"In my candidacy at the White Institute in the early fifties, I was interviewed by Dr. Thompson, took her courses, was in supervision with her and later came to know her during summers on the Cape. I am delighted to see this thoughtful and respectful book by Dr. D'Ercole. It is a labor of love by a prominent feminist psychoanalyst in tribute to a much-overlooked major contributor to psychoanalytic theory and practice. That is, of course, consistent with the treatment of women in most scientific venues at the time, but also 'Clara's' (we all called her that, but not always to her face) modesty led her to act as a portal to the work of Sullivan and Fromm—the two other founders of WAW. Dr. D'Ercole has done an outstanding job of explicating Dr. Thompson's prescient contributions to modern psychoanalytic theory and practice but has also grasped her in her most human aspects. For all my long association with Dr. Thompson, and in spite of her friendliness and egalitarianism, I hardly knew her. I trust this outstanding book will remedy this oversight and revitalize a much-deserved interest in this most interesting and complex person."

Edgar Levenson is a fellow emeritus, faculty, training, and supervisory analyst at the William Alanson White Institute; he is adjunct clinical professor of Psychology at New York University, and author of *Fallacy of Understanding; The Ambiguity of Change; The Purloined Self;* and *Interpersonal Psychoanalysis and the Enigma of Consciousness*

"Clara Thompson was not only one of the most important leaders in the psychoanalysis of her time, but also one of the singular figures in the entire history of the discipline. She was a pioneer in so many ways, founding and then directing one of the most significant psychoanalytic institutes, bringing together the work of Erich Fromm and Harry Stack Sullivan to create interpersonal psychoanalysis, and creating one of the first bodies of work devoted to the psychology of women. She was one of those who created the study of gender and sexuality. She was a powerfully inspiring leader at a time when that was highly unusual for a woman in psychiatry or psychoanalysis. Thompson richly deserves Ann D'Ercole's deep, thorough, and moving account of her life. This two-volume work is absolutely riveting, an instant classic that will be read and studied not only by psychoanalysts and other psychotherapists, but by anyone interested in cultural history, feminism, the history of psychiatry, and gender and sexuality."

Donnel Stern most recently authored *The Infinity of the Unsaid: Unformulated Experience, Language, and the Nonverbal*

"Ann D'Ercole's two-volume biography carefully documents and reveals Clara Thompson's often-overlooked role and contributions to the development of interpersonal psychoanalysis in the United States. 'Clara,' as interpersonalists still refer to her today, was analyzed by Sándor Ferenczi in Budapest and worked closely with Harry Stack Sullivan, Erich Fromm and Frieda Fromm-Reichman. She was the first Director of the William Alanson White Institute in New York City (currently housed in the Clara Thompson building) and the training and supervising analyst for many pioneers of contemporary interpersonal and relational theory. D'Ercole has done an exemplary and engaging job of correcting this historical omission of Thompson's foundational role as 'An American Psychoanalyst.'"

Jack Drescher is a training and supervising analyst at the William Alanson White Institute; adjunct professor of the Postdoctoral Program in Psychotherapy and Psychoanalysis; a clinical professor of Psychiatry at Columbia University; and senior psychoanalytic consultant at the Columbia Center for Psychoanalytic Training and Research

"Ann D'Ercole has accomplished a special scholarly work about Clara Thompson, M.D. Has Thompson having been a foremost student of Sándor Ferenczi placed her in the analytic shadows? Ann's thorough, lively and insightful writing brings Thompson out of the shadows and into the limelight where she belongs. Ann's outstanding research has clarified Thompson's brilliant contributions to psychoanalysis: a prominent figure in establishing the American School of Psychoanalysis; a leading contributor in the formation of the Interpersonal School of Psychoanalysis; a leading student and advocate of the work of Sándor Ferenczi and Henry Stack Sullivan; a founder of the William Alanson White Institute; a leading feminist of her time; a pioneering theorist and clinician in establishing the two person perspective in psychoanalysis. Ann's biography of Thompson should become the premium resource that rediscovers the importance of Clara Thompson for psychoanalysis."

Arnold Wm. Rachman is a Training and Supervisory Analyst, Postgraduate Psychoanalytic Institute, NYC; Clinical Professor of Psychology, Adelphi University Postdoctoral Program in Psychoanalysis and Psychotherapy, Garden City, NY; Associate Professor of Psychiatry, New York University Medical Center, NYC; Donor, Elizabeth Severn Papers, The Library of Congress; recent publication - *Psychoanalysis and Society's Neglect of the Sexual Abuse of the Children, Youth and Adults*, Routledge

"In this engaging paean to the life of Clara Thompson, D'Ercole excavates, brings to life, and carries forth the historical record in adroitly making the case that Thompson deserves placement in the upper echelons of the pantheon of psychoanalysts. She plumbs the depths of her own personal connection to Thompson in illuminating the essential contributions of Thompson to the field of interpersonal psychoanalysis. A hidden gem, not just for readers unfamiliar with Thompson's work, this is a must read for all."

Jean Petrucelli is faculty, training, and supervising analyst at the William Alanson White Institute; adjunct professor and clinical consultant of the NYU Postdoctoral Program in Psychotherapy and Psychoanalysis; and most recently, co-editor of the book *Patriarchy and Its Discontents*

Clara M. Thompson's Early Years and Professional Awakening

In the first of this two-volume biography, Ann D'Ercole tells the story of Clara M. Thompson, drawing extensively on unpublished archival interviews and correspondence, to provide a full and complex picture of an early American pioneer of psychoanalysis.

The book begins by exploring Thompson's youth, which was steeped in evangelical Christianity, and conveys the difficulty that Thompson experienced as she resisted the restrictive conventions of femininity prevalent at the time. Despite this, Thompson's talent as a student continually shines through, as D'Ercole gives readers an account of Thompson's life at the Johns Hopkins School of Medicine, where she would work alongside the innovative psychiatrist Adolf Meyer. Thompson's ground-breaking theoretical and clinical achievements continue to be celebrated, as D'Ercole explores Thompson's life-changing experiences whilst in psychoanalytic treatment with Sándor Ferenczi.

By allowing her voice to prevail, this book recognizes Thompson's vital work in the formulation of interpersonal psychoanalysis, rendering it invaluable for interpersonal psychoanalysts wishing to understand Thompson's role in the development of the school.

Ann D'Ercole is a Clinical Associate Professor of Psychology at the New York University Postdoctoral Program in Psychotherapy and Psychoanalysis, where she is both teaching faculty and supervisor. She is also a distinguished visiting faculty at the William Alanson White Institute and recipient of the APA, Division 39, Sexualities and Gender Identities Award for Outstanding Contributions to the Advancement of Sexualities and Gender Identities in Psychoanalysis. Dr. D'Ercole is in private practice in New York City.

Psychoanalysis in A New Key Book Series
Donnel Stern
Series Editor

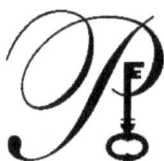

When music is played in a new key, the melody does not change, but the notes that make up the composition do: change in the context of continuity, continuity that perseveres through change. Psychoanalysis in a New Key publishes books that share the aims psychoanalysts have always had, but that approach them differently. The books in the series are not expected to advance any particular theoretical agenda, although to this date most have been written by analysts from the Interpersonal and Relational orientations.

The most important contribution of a psychoanalytic book is the communication of something that nudges the reader's grasp of clinical theory and practice in an unexpected direction. Psychoanalysis in a New Key creates a deliberate focus on innovative and unsettling clinical thinking. Because that kind of thinking is encouraged by exploration of the sometimes surprising contributions to psychoanalysis of ideas and findings from other fields, Psychoanalysis in a New Key particularly encourages interdisciplinary studies. Books in the series have married psychoanalysis with dissociation, trauma theory, sociology, and criminology. The series is open to the consideration of studies examining the relationship between psychoanalysis and any other field—for instance, biology, literary and art criticism, philosophy, systems theory, anthropology, and political theory.

But innovation also takes place within the boundaries of psychoanalysis, and Psychoanalysis in a New Key therefore also presents work that reformulates thought and practice without leaving the precincts of the field. Books in the series focus, for example, on the significance of personal values in psychoanalytic practice, on the complex interrelationship between the analyst's clinical work and personal life, on the consequences for the clinical situation when patient and analyst are from different cultures, and on the need for psychoanalysts to accept the degree to which they knowingly satisfy their own wishes during treatment hours, often to the patient's detriment. A full list of all titles in this series is available at:

www.routledge.com/Psychoanalysis-in-a-New-Key-Book-Series/book-series/LEAPNKBS

Clara M. Thompson's Early Years and Professional Awakening

An American Psychoanalyst
(1893-1933)

Ann D'Ercole

Routledge
Taylor & Francis Group

LONDON AND NEW YORK

Cover image: "Dr. Clara Thompson" by Lotte Jacobi. *University of New Hampshire*. Used with permission. © 2022 The University of New Hampshire.

First published 2023
by Routledge
4 Park Square, Milton Park, Abingdon, Oxon OX14 4RN

and by Routledge
605 Third Avenue, New York, NY 10158

Routledge is an imprint of the Taylor & Francis Group, an informa business

© 2023 Ann D'Ercole

The right of Ann D'Ercole to be identified as author of this work has been asserted in accordance with sections 77 and 78 of the Copyright, Designs and Patents Act 1988.

British Library Cataloguing-in-Publication Data
A catalogue record for this book is available from the British Library

Library of Congress Cataloging-in-Publication Data
Names: D'Ercole, Ann, author.
Title: Clara M. Thompson's early years and professional awakening: an American psychoanalyst (1893-1933) / Ann D'Ercole.
Description: Abingdon, Oxon ; New York, NY : Routledge, 2023. | Includes bibliographical references and index.
Identifiers: LCCN 2022016960 (print) | LCCN 2022016961 (ebook) | ISBN 9781032199955 (hardback) | ISBN 9781032199979 (paperback) | ISBN 9781003261797 (ebook)
Subjects: LCSH: Thompson, Clara, 1893–1958. | Psychiatrists— United States—Biography. | Psychoanalysts—United States— Biography. | Psychoanalysis.
Classification: LCC RC438.6.T556 D468 2023 (print) | LCC RC438.6.T556 (ebook) | DDC 616.89/17092 [B]—dc23/eng/20220713
LC record available at https://lccn.loc.gov/2022016960
LC ebook record available at https://lccn.loc.gov/2022016961

Every effort has been made to contact copyright-holders. Please advise the publisher of any errors or omissions, and these will be corrected in subsequent editions.

ISBN: 978-1-032-19995-5 (hbk)
ISBN: 978-1-032-19997-9 (pbk)
ISBN: 978-1-003-26179-7 (ebk)

DOI: 10.4324/9781003261797

Typeset in Times New Roman
by Apex CoVantage, LLC

For Linda, Tony, David, Laura, Marci, Helen, Andrew, Kaley, Frida and Ryder.

Contents

Acknowledgments

There are so many individuals and institutions that made this book possible. Before thanking them, I want to say something about what it was like to do this work. Doing the research was absorbing and gratifying; the writing was more difficult. Writing is always hard.

Well into the project, SARS-COV-2 descended on the world and sent me into isolation for what is now nearly two years. The virus brought fears and worries; I was privileged to isolate in Truro with my partner, and our dog Bear. It was comforting having one of my sons and two of my grandchildren nearby, though our visits were limited to outside and wearing masks. This unprecedented situation allowed me to work on the project almost without interruption. Living through a pandemic was something else I came to share with Clara Thompson.

This biography developed over years with many conversations with other psychoanalysts. I especially thank Dr. Edgar Levenson for his wise counsel and continuing support. His recollections and firsthand perspective have been an important influence. In 2018 I met, at Dr. Lewis Aron's suggestion, Dr. Arnold Rachman, an expert on both Sándor Ferenczi's work and Ferenczi's patient, Elizabeth Severn. He was a muse who read drafts and provided valuable comments. He shared my excitement for the work. I am deeply grateful.

My choice to begin Thompson's biography near the end of her career with her interview for the Freud Archive I attribute to Justin Kaplan, the American writer and winner of both the National Book Award and, in 1967, the Pulitzer Prize. I met Kaplan in his writing course at the Truro Center for the Arts at Castle Hill. He argued for something that challenged my psychoanalytic perspective on early childhood: "Everyone has a childhood; life does not get interesting until people start making decisions." I came to value his perspective. You can understand much about a person through their decisions.

Support for the project came from many additional directions, including from my study group on Interpersonal Psychoanalysis (before COVID-19 sent us into isolation). It included Drs. Lynn Passy, Forbes Singer, Brenda Tepper, Catherine Baker-Pitts, and William Auerbach. My friends and colleagues, Anita Herron, Martin Devine, Linda Brady, Barbara Suter, Jack Drescher, Lewis Friedman, Judith Alpert, Nina Thomas, Arnold Rachman, and Kenneth Eisold, read drafts and provided comments. Dr. Nellie Thompson, Curator, Archives & Special Collections, A.A. Brill Library/NYPSI, generously shared information and read a draft of a chapter. She introduced me to the work of Dr. Elizabeth Capelle. Capelle's (1993) dissertation in history traces important aspects of Clara Thompson's life. Her extensive research illuminated the role of Thompson's involvement with the Free Will Baptists, her incisive comments on Thompson's early identifications as well as the critical feminist contributions made by Thompson add significantly to this narrative. I thank her for allowing me to quote widely from her work.

Christopher Busa, Peter Manso, and Anton Van Dereck Haunstrup helped to fill in details of life in Provincetown. Stephen Magliocco shared his architect's view of the memorials to Clara Thompson and Henry Major in the Provincetown Cemetery (discussed in Volume 2).

I thank Richard Herman, Director of Administration at William Alanson White (WAW), and Elizabeth Rodman, Administrative Manager, who made the archive at WAW available to me. Dr. Marylou Lionells, a former director of the William Alanson White Institute and co-editor of the *Handbook of Interpersonal Psychoanalysis*, graciously offered helpful comments and questions. Dr. Kenneth Eisold, esteemed author and current President of the Board at WAW, offered his support, read a chapter, and provided valuable comments. I am enormously grateful to Dr. Judith Dupont for helping to clarify notations in the Clinical Diary of Sándor Ferenczi. She thoughtfully and graciously responded to my questions about Ferenczi's *Clinical Diary*, clarifying some confusions Arnold Rachman and I had about specific entries.

The New York University Postdoctoral Program in Psychotherapy and Psychoanalysis (NYU Postdoc), my primary affiliation, is a generative community that fostered and encouraged this biography's necessity. Two past directors of the program are no doubt represented in these pages for their encouragement and foresight. Dr. Bernie Kalinkowitz, former Postdoc director, was a patient of Clara Thompson's. Dr. Lewis Aron, a former director, was sadly too ill to participate in the project, but he encouraged me to proceed. Lew was very interested in Clara Thompson's relationship to Izette de Forest and their complicated feelings towards their fellow patient Elizabeth Severn. I hope I have begun to open up those feelings in the chapters.

I am grateful to Donnel Stern, founder and editor of the Routledge series "Psychoanalysis in a New Key," for including this biography in the series.

I thank Dr. Louis Rose, Executive Director, Sigmund Freud Archives, and Dr. Emanuel Garcia, Kurt Eissler's literary executor, for allowing the 1954 interview to be reprinted in its entirety "without editorial emendations, typographical corrections, deletions, altered punctuation, or ellipses."

The Graduate Society of the Postdoctoral Program generously provided me with two Scholar's Grants that helped to support the project. They also furnished a forum for presenting this work early in its development.

I thank The Alan Mason Chesney Medical Archives of the Johns Hopkins Medical Institutions, specifically Marjorie W. Kehoe, Reference and Accessioning Archivist, who helped find the materials I requested. Likewise, Marisa Shaari at the DeWitt Wallace Institute for the History of Psychiatry & the Oskar Diethelm Library at Weill Cornell Medical College assisted in locating papers and correspondence. Librarians are critical to projects like this one. They reach out to other institutions and share generously. I thank them all. A special thank you to Dr. Rainer Funk, of the Literary Estate of Erich Fromm, Erich Fromm Institute, Tübingen, for sending me an invaluable collection of the Fromm and Thompson correspondence and for allowing me to quote from some of those letters.

During the project, I sought out and received editorial assistance from Adrienne Hall, Anne Ranson, Kristopher Spring, and Kim Berstein and assistance from Georgina Cutterbuck at Routledge Press. Each helped with different phases of the project and helped make the text flow smoothly, structuring it for publication.

My partner, Linda Brady, encouraged, supported, and brought her perceptive questions to me as she read and edited each chapter. Her enthusiasm and support gave me the confidence to continue.

My family is a part of this book, too. Indeed, my mother, Rose Marion Iorio D'Ercole, a 20th-century woman, would have delighted in the fact of this book. My father, Raymond D'Ercole, died way too early as a misdiagnosed dementia patient. I am thankful that psychiatric research has improved the treatment and care of early dementia patients. My sons Tony and David, my daughter Laura, and my daughters-in-law Marci and Helen supported and encouraged me to stay the course. I appreciated Laura's insights as a professor of sociology along the way. My granddaughters Kaley and Frida are excellent storytellers and writers. I hope they like this one. I appreciated Kaley's help with edits and our lunches at Terralucci. My grandson Andrew read and offered valuable comments early in the writing. Thank you to my grandson Ryder for opening my eyes to what is culturally relevant now.

This book is also about all the psychoanalytic partners, patients, and analysts who undertake the treacherous and enormously gratifying journey of self-discovery. In that way, we are all pioneers.

Credits List

The author gratefully acknowledges the permission provided to republish the following materials:

- Analytic Observations during a course of a manic-depressive psychosis, Clara Thompson (ed.), *The Psychoanalytic Review*, 17(2). Republished with permission of Guilford Publications, Inc. © 1913; permission conveyed through Copyright Clearance Center, Inc.
- Audio material from Pembroke Center Oral History Collection, OH.1s.2013.002, Christine Dunlap Farnham Archive, Brown University Library.
- Clara Thompson, M.D. Interviewed by K. R. Eissler, M.D. June 4, 1952. Courtesy of Dr. Emanuel E. Garcia, the literary executor of the K.R. Eissler Estate, and Louis Rose, Executive Director, Sigmund Freud Archives. Sigmund Freud Papers: Interviews and Recollections, Set A, 1914–1998 (Box 122). Manuscripts Division, Library of Congress, Washington, DC. www.loc.gov/item/mss3999001575/
- "Concepts of the Self in Interpersonal Theory", Clara Thompson, *American Journal of* Psychotherapy 12(1), pp. 5–17. Reprinted with permission from the *American Journal of Psychotherapy* (Copyright © 1958). American Psychiatric Association. All Rights Reserved.
- Documents and photographic material from the archive of the William Alanson White Institute, as provided by Richard Herman, Director of Administration at the Institute.
- Documents and correspondence from The Alan Mason Chesney Medical Archives, The Johns Hopkins University, The Johns Hopkins Hospital.

- THE CLINICAL DIARY OF SÁNDOR FERENCZI by Sándor Ferenczi, edited by Judith Dupont, translated by Michael Balint and Nicola Zarday Jackson, Cambridge, MA: Harvard University Press, Copyright © 1985, 1988 by Payot, Paris, by arrangement with Mark Paterson; English translation Copyright © 1985, 1988 by Nicola Jackson. Used by permission. All rights reserved.
- Dutiful Child Resistance, Clara Thompson, *The Psychoanalytic Review*, pp. 426–433. Republished with permission of Guilford Publications, Inc. © 1943; permission conveyed through Copyright Clearance Center, Inc.
- Ferenczi's Forgotten Messenger: The Life and Work of Izette de Forest, B. W. Brennan, *American Imago*, 66(4). Republished with permission of Johns Hopkins University Press—Journals © 2009; permission conveyed through Copyright Clearance Center, Inc. URL: http://call iope.jhu.edu/journals/american%5Fimago
- Frosch, J., The New York Psychoanalytic Civil War. *Journal of the American Psychoanalytic Association* (39:4), pp. 1037–1064, Copyright © 1991 (Taylor & Francis). Reprinted by Permission of SAGE Publications.
- Photographic material and correspondence reprinted courtesy of the Oskar Diethelm Library, DeWitt Wallace Institute of Psychiatry: History, Policy, & the Arts, Weill Cornell Medical College.
- Thompson, C., Notes on the Psychoanalytic Significance of the Choice of Analyst. *Psychiatry* (1:2), Copyright © 1938 The Washington School of Psychiatry (www.wspdc.org). Reprinted by permission of Informa UK Limited, trading as Taylor & Francis Group, www.tandfonline.com on behalf of www.wspdc.org.
- Thompson, C., The Role of Women in this Culture. *Psychiatry* (4:1), copyright © 1941 The Washington School of Psychiatry (www.wspdc.org). Reprinted by permission of Informa UK Limited, trading as Taylor & Francis Group, www.tandfonline.com on behalf of www.wspdc.org.
- From *Interpersonal Psychoanalysis* by W. Grant Thompson, Copyright © 1964. Reprinted by permission of Basic Books, an imprint of Hachette Book Group, Inc.

Timeline of Key Events

Born Providence, RI 1893

Total Immersion Baptism September 29, 1905

Announces during Christian Endeavor meeting intension to become a
    medical missionary 1908

Classical High School 1908–1912

Pembroke/Brown University 1912–1916

Danvers State Hospital, for premedical school work 1915–1916

Johns Hopkins Medical School 1916–1920

St. Elizabeth Hospital summer of 1917—meets William Alanson White,
    Edward J. Kempf, and Joseph (Snake) Thompson

House Medical Officer, Johns Hopkins 1920–1921

Rotating Internship at NY Infirmary for Women and Children 1921

Residency 3 years—Phipps Clinic, Adolf Meyer, Director 1922–1924

Assistant resident in psychiatry 1922–1925; begins psychoanalytic treat-
    ment with Joseph Thompson

Instructor in Psychiatry at Johns Hopkins 1923–1925

Meets Harry Stack Sullivan 1923

Break with Adolf Meyer 1925

Begins private practice 1925

Meets Sándor Ferenczi at The New School in NYC 1927

Teaches mental hygiene at Institute of Euthenics at Vassar College
    1928–1929

Travels to Budapest in the summers for psychoanalysis with Sándor Fer-
    enczi 1928, 1929, 1930

President Wash/Bal Society 1930

Death of Thompson's Father 1930 (mother died 1952)

Miracle Club 1930–1931

Moves to Budapest to finish her analysis June 1931–1933

Thompson attends 12th International Psychoanalytic Congress, Wiesbaden, in September (1932) where Ferenczi read The passions of adults and their influence on the sexual and character development of children (1933). Published originally in German, Ferenczi, S. (1934) Gedanken über das Trauma: Aus dem Nachlaß von. Internationale Zeitschrift für Psychoanalyse 20:5–12; and then as, Ferenczi, S. (1949) Confusion of tongues between adults and children: the language of tenderness and passion. International *Journal of Psychoanalysis*, 30, 225–230; and as, Ferenczi, S. (1988) Confusion of Tongues between Adults and the Child, Contemporary Psychoanalysis, 24:2, 196–206, DOI: 10.1080/00107530.1988.10746234 *Int. Z. f. Psa*, 19–5 (German original). Confusion of the tongues between the adults and the child (The language of tenderness and of passion) (1949). *International Journal of Psychoanalysis, 30*, 225–230 (English translation).

Death of Sándor Ferenczi May 23, 1933

Returns to US 1933

Introduction

Beginnings and Endings

I chose to begin the biography of Clara M. Thompson near the end of her life. It allows for an appreciation of the depth of her experience and the breadth of her perspective in the developing field of psychoanalysis. It is 1952; she is being interviewed by Dr. Kurt Eissler for the Freud Archives. I invite you to imagine an opening scene with her seated across from Eissler in a mid-century modern-appointed office overlooking Central Park. Bookshelves are prominently featured.

Beginning here provided an opportunity to hear Clara Thompson recount a segment of the history of psychoanalysis as she witnessed its evolution. With permission from the Kurt Eissler Estate, the interview is reprinted in its complete form taking advantage of an opportunity to bring this moment in the past into the present. Thompson (1938) advises that in the study of any phenomenon in psychoanalysis, "meaning often attaches to subtleties." This interview reminds us how subtleties are difficult to capture and at times difficult to decipher. Fortunately, the interview has been preserved and available for us to continually consider.

This first volume of the biography of Thompson centers on her early life experiences, and professional awakening (1893–1933). Thompson grew up in an era when the struggle for freedoms—religious, racial, women's, and worker's rights—were gaining ground. It was a time of opportunity for white Americans in Thompson's hometown, the industrial seaport city of Providence, Rhode Island. Individual self-realization was promoted as a means of meeting the needs of the community as well as the self. These were driving forces in American culture at the beginning of the 20th century. In many ways, it was both a time of great thinkers who spoke to the social and cultural transformations to come and a time of an America built on myths and symbols, like the idea of new England.

DOI: 10.4324/9781003261797-1

Living as Clara Thompson did in a large extended family where familial dynamics were rife with tension influenced her development. As a child, she learned to disguise her true feelings in what she later came to describe as a defensive compliance. It allowed a way to get along with the adults, particularly her mother. Her maternal side of the family was very religious while the paternal side was less observant. Thompson's values were instilled within the practices of the Free Will Baptists, the religious community of her parents. She was raised to believe that life demanded responsibility and came with a mission, and that importantly not one's "color nor sex" should impose a barrier. Her mother was stern and abusive. Her father was ambitious and focused on his career though she was his favorite.

Throughout her childhood, Thompson was an excellent student and popular with other children. She attended the best secondary school in the area and by then had professed her aspiration to become a medical missionary.

While at Pembroke College/Brown University, she cast aside all spiritual beliefs and their confining gendered demands and instead embraced a set of values that set her own moral compass. She trained to become a psychiatrist at Johns Hopkins School of Medicine under the tutelage of Adolf Meyer and William Alanson White. In 1923 during her residency, she met Harry Stack Sullivan. It was an unusual beginning. She had presented her first paper while suffering from typhoid fever. Sullivan was taken with her immediately. He did not know she was running a high temperature and thought instead that she might be schizophrenic. They established a lasting and influential relationship. Both Thompson and Sullivan wanted the world to be changed for the better and for people's lives to be improved. It was a 20th-century American dream and a psychoanalytic aspiration.

Thompson made stunning life choices: she chose a career over marriage, and she decided to become a physician when medical schools admitted few women. She sailed aboard a steamship to Europe choosing to undergo psychoanalytic treatment with Sándor Ferenczi, a favored disciple of Sigmund Freud. She became a psychoanalyst when very few analysts existed in the United States and even fewer were women. Romantically she was rumored to have lesbian relationships and that she was bisexual. In her mid-forties, she chose to have an unconventional relationship with a married man who was only partially available.

This biography leans toward an oral history tradition, as it features, when possible, Thompson's voice—in her interviews, correspondence, and scholarly essays. It is supplemented at times by her friends' and colleagues' testimonials to capture her life story from different perspectives. The story offers a richly layered portrait of a daring woman, a psychoanalyst in the field's early days. The narrative fills historical gaps as it corrects and updates the record of Thompson's theoretical contributions and her role in the development of psychoanalysis. Her history is presented with all her complexities and contradictions, leaving room for not knowing. After all, there is still much we don't know about Clara Thompson. In telling the story of her life, certain aspects of the historical development of psychoanalysis are illuminated, featuring a cast of early psychoanalysts like Izette de Forest and Elizabeth Severn who have yet to receive their due attention.

Every life story is more than the sum of birth, education, career, relationships, and death; rather how these life events have shaped the individual and, in the case of Clara Thompson, including her legacy of scholarly contributions is paramount. This provides an opportunity to understand Clara Thompson the person and to consider how and why her theoretical concepts and clinical work took the shape they did. It allows us to pay homage to a formidable legacy that gives weight to the assertion that she is the architect of the American Interpersonal Tradition rather than the men (Sullivan and Fromm) who most often receive the credit.

Before beginning this project, I had not considered writing a biography, though I did write two psychohistorical studies of two of Freud's cases (D'Ercole & Waxenberg, 1999; D'Ercole, 1999). My graduate degree in Community Psychology from New York University was followed by the Postdoctoral Program in Psychiatric Epidemiology at Columbia University. I began my professional career conducting research on the homeless populations in New York City. By using a version of the life history method in my research, I was unknowingly following the path of the early psychoanalytic pioneers who were influenced by the culture and personality school and methods of anthropologists. My work was published in 1990 (D'Ercole & Struening) and in a *Special Issue of the American Psychologist* in 1991 (Milburn & D'Ercole, 1991a; 1991b).

My turn toward psychoanalysis evolved over the course of my own therapeutic experiences. I embarked on psychoanalytic training at the New York University Postdoctoral Program in Psychotherapy and Psychoanalysis where I found a community of like-minded people interested in viewing individual problems through the lens of culture.

In 1993 I traveled to the first conference on Ferenczi's work held in Budapest, "The Talking Therapy: Ferenczi and the Psychoanalytic Vocation." During that trip, I visited Ferenczi's house in the swanky suburbs of Budapest. I opened the gate and walked into the backyard garden as Thompson might have done when she saw him. I took photos of the house and garden. I had in mind capturing something of these historic figures, though I had not yet thought of writing Thompson's biography. I had visited Freud's homes both in Vienna and London, but the connection I felt to Ferenczi's gracious residence was different. Ferenczi was more approachable than Freud. Am I romanticizing the experience?

My autobiographical account of growing up in an immigrant Italian family (D'Ercole, 2012) perhaps gave me the courage to undertake this biography. Many have asked me, "Why Clara Thompson, what drew you to her?" There is no simple answer to that question. It was clear to me that Thompson was an underrecognized pioneering psychoanalyst in the history of the field. Her story needed telling. Her steps in the 20th century toward sexual and racial theorizing are both praiseworthy and sometimes disappointing. As I began the project, I wondered with trepidation, how does one write a biography of a 20th-century psychoanalytic pioneer who you never met?

My transgenerational connections to Clara Thompson were certainly influential in my choice to write this biography. Those connections distinguish me as a psychoanalytic granddaughter of Clara Thompson. They include my analyst Edgar Levenson who early in his career was in supervision with Clara Thompson for two years. He encouraged me to simultaneously value curiosity and character. He cultivated an interest in what is being avoided and or disguised and how the analyst is as much a part of the clinical action as the patient. My clinical consultant, Benjamin Wolstein, an analysand of Thompson's, taught me something he learned from Clara Thompson about connecting with what he called the psychic center of the self, an emotionally intense and genuine connection that influenced my clinical practice. My analyst, Esther Menaker, spoke fondly of Clara Thompson. Esther Menaker, like Clara Thompson, was one of those courageous women who traveled to Europe to undergo psychoanalysis in its earliest days. In Esther's case, she chose Vienna in the late 1920s and Anna Freud as her analyst (Menaker, 1989). My training years were populated with analysts who either were in analysis with Clara Thompson or were supervised by her.

While not formally trained as a psychoanalyst, Annilese Reiss had a major impact on my life. I saw her for treatment during my college and graduate school years. She encouraged me to follow my interest in psychoanalysis. Reiss was a survivor. She escaped Nazi Germany by walking to Italy. Her fondness for all things Italian matched mine. She had been an assistant to Rene Spitz in his studies of unmothered infants who experience a failure to thrive. She was also very fond of Bernard Kalinkowitz, Thompson's analysand, and spoke of him often. I met Bernie when he was the Director of the clinical psychology program at NYU. Our connection was renewed when I entered NYU Postdoctoral Program in Psychotherapy and Psychoanalysis for psychoanalytic training. Through Bernie my connection to Clara Thompson and the Interpersonalists continued. These threads of psychoanalytic filiations create a family tree in psychoanalysis (Falzeder, 2015). My family tree has many branches that connect and interconnect with Clara Thompson.

Another link with Thompson came to me close to home when I discovered that Thompson's summer house on Commercial Street in Provincetown was a stone's throw from my summer home in North Truro. Knowing we walked the same paths on the Outer Cape seemed to cement my connection. Thompson was a woman who appreciated the seclusion of the outer Cape filled with its art, ideas, and unconventional people.

Though my journey into the field was different than these early pioneering, rebellious first-generation analysts, I had my share of adventures—encounter groups, primal scream therapy, gestalt therapy. I date my relationship with psychoanalysis to the day when I found Freud's *Interpretation of Dreams* in my local public library at the age of twelve. Despite my curiosity in the book, one I thought held answers to my questions about sex and gender, it was decades before I resumed my interest. Like many in my generation, my feminist awakening came during the late 1960s and 1970s, a time of considerable turmoil and personal and cultural upheaval. Like Clara Thompson, my college experience opened my eyes to things that I had not seen or allowed myself to feel. I strongly identify with her rebellion. My first-generational status as a daughter of an Italian immigrant family provided an outsider's perspective on the role of the dominant culture.

In this volume, we come to know Clara Thompson as she developed and evolved into a young professional woman. Her story tells us something of her journey from the confines of a religious upbringing to what it was like to become a psychoanalyst in the early days of the 20th century.

This narrative comes with a warning: consensus—even for things observed at the moment, let alone decades later—is impossible. Stories like this one are always a process and subject to change as more information and different perspectives are added. By definition, a biography accounts for someone's life written by someone else, the biographer is always attending to some details while passing over others.

My Process

In the course of my research on Clara Thompson I contacted the institutions she attended, hoping to discover her correspondence. At the Alan Mason Chesney Medical Archives of Johns Hopkins Medicine, Nursing, and Public Health there were two letters referenced below that were in the Adolf Meyer collection 1890–1940. I discovered correspondence held at the DeWitt Wallace Institute for the History of Psychiatry & the Oskar Diethelm Library, Weill Cornell Medical College, within Ralph Crowley's papers. These findings included a stash of handwritten letters that enrich and contextualize the telling of Thompson's life by admitting her voice into the historical data. I searched for letters between Sullivan and Thompson and found none but I did find important correspondence between Thompson and her third analyst, Erich Fromm. Those letters were shared with me courtesy of Rainer Funk, Erich Fromm Archive, Tübingen.

The Clinical Diary of Sándor Ferenczi (Dupont, 1988) provided valuable and confounding information concerning her psychoanalytic treatment with Ferenczi in Budapest. I focus closely on the entries that relate to Thompson to find her voice in their collaborative work.

Maurice Green (1964a) authored a significant thirty-page biographical essay titled "Her Life" that he tucked at the end of the volume he edited of her collected papers definitively titled, *Interpersonal Psychoanalysis: The Selected Papers of Clara M. Thompson* (1964b). The relevance of his choice of that title for the volume is a leitmotif in this biography; that is, he installed Clara Thompson as the leader of Interpersonal Psychoanalysis. His biographical essay is the backbone of information on Clara Thompson's life. He had the advantage of knowing her and was also able to interview other people who knew her, so when he writes that Thompson could be both warm and attentive and detached and private, we understand his assertions came from his personal experience. Green, who was her analysand and student, no doubt he felt a deep sense of gratitude and affection for her. He described her as having a sense of humor and an affectionate smile, which led others to expect more openness and vulnerability. These contradictions were influenced by both the New England culture where she grew up and the rigid religious community of her youth. For decades, Green's essay stood as the definitive biography of Clara M. Thompson. However, its brevity left great swaths of her life in the shadows, while preserving her significant work.

I have drawn from Elizabeth Capelle's (1993, 1998) deep dive into the Free Will Baptist religious community and Thompson's early aspiration to become a medical missionary to expand the understanding of that influential aspect of her life. Capelle's analysis of Thompson's place in the history of feminism and as a cultural psychoanalyst has been invaluable.

Writing this biography has been a continual series of beginnings. First there was the person, Clara M. Thompson, whose essays on the psychology of women I encountered during my college years. Her critiques of Freud's views on women were more in line with my budding sense of the role of culture in human development. Later as a psychoanalytic candidate, two of my supervisors were Thompson's analysands, Ruth Lesser and Benjamin Wolstein. It was Benjamin Wolstein who spoke most about Thompson's influence on him. I first read *The Clinical Diary of Sándor Ferenczi* (Dupont, 1988) with Benjamin Wolstein. It was with Wolstein that my first conversation developed over the delayed publication of the *Clinical Diary*.

I think it is fair to say that Wolstein adored Clara Thompson. He told me that at the end of his analysis with her, he gave her a string of pearls which she loved. It reminded me of the gifts Freud gave to his close circle of disciples. Wolstein continued his story adding that when Thompson was dying, she asked to be buried wearing those pearls. It was a touching sign of their enduring connection and a stark anthesis to the cool detached psychoanalyst mostly promoted in popular culture.

Stories like these can get lost when the storyteller dies unless someone carries it forward. This is one of the critical functions of the oral history tradition. Recounting history is imperiled by death, fading memory, amnesia, and nostalgia. In the case of rebels or dissidents, an imposed silencing can create a fracture in knowledge about the past. I hope this story of the trailblazing Clara Thompson remedies that rupture.

There is a loneliness that seems to haunt the story of Clara M. Thompson. At times she was deeply depressed. She first sought psychoanalytic treatment during her psychiatric residency hoping no doubt to rid herself of those dark feelings. Her second analyst was Sándor Ferenczi. The *Clinical Diary of Sándor Ferenczi* (Dupont, 1988) states that Clara Thompson had been "grossly sexually abused by her father" (p. 3). That entry surprised Wolstein and many others. He questioned its veracity. Chapter 4 investigates the assertion of sexual abuse and concludes that the mixing of patients in the *Clinical Diary* in order to maintain the privacy of patients complicates what can be known.

Interviews

Those who knew Clara Thompson, and those who only heard about her, universally referred to her by her given name, Clara. I found this to be true, especially at William Alanson White Institute, where she served as Director. The choice of the informal may indicate something about the intimacy and affection bestowed on her. Yet, we rarely hear Sigmund Freud or Sándor Ferenczi referred to by their given names, suggesting that the use of an honorific title (Mr., Ms., Dr., etc.) or surname comes with a gendered bias. I refer to Clara Thompson throughout this book mostly in a formal way, using her full name or her surname; admittedly having spent so much time researching her life I too often refer to her as "Clara."

Here Today, Gone Tomorrow

Thompson was a prominent figure during the 1930s, 1940s, and 1950s, then she disappeared from the analytic canon. Understanding the breadth of her scholarly contributions entails a mission of discovery, since many articles are not easily found on the usual search engines. Where possible, I have quoted from the original publications; when that was not possible, the edited volume of her work assembled by Maurice Green was relied upon.

Thompson's essays are discussed as they inform us about her personality as well as her professional evolution. She built a bridge between Sándor Ferenczi and Adolf Meyer, between Europe and America. There are side trips into the analytic siblings of Clara Thompson in Budapest who were also early contributors to the field.

The process of writing this biography has been a continual series of beginnings involving uncovering information that elaborated her story which evolved into two volumes covering the years 1893–1933 and 1933–1958.

In some ways, this biography began on May 23, 1961, when Dr. Maurice Green wrote a letter to the Registrar at Johns Hopkins Medical School. He explained that he was engaged in writing a biographical and historical introduction to the collected papers of Clara M. Thompson, MD (Johns Hopkins, 1920; Phipps resident, 1920–1923; Instructor in Psychiatry, 1923–1925).

He writes,

I would very much appreciate any information you can give me regarding her academic and clinical education. In addition, I would appreciate any information you can give regarding the courses taught by Taneyhill in the History of Psychoanalysis in America. Were there any other courses or lectures in psychoanalysis during that decade (1916–1925)? Did Herbert S. Jennings teach in the medical school?

Sincerely,

Maurice R. Green, MD

On June 23, 1961, Mary E. Burke, Registrar at Hopkins, replied:

Dear Dr. Green:

This is in reply to your letter of May 23, 1961, requesting information about Dr. Clara M. Thompson.

Dr. Thompson received an A.B. degree from Brown University on June 21, 1916 and the M.D. degree from the Johns Hopkins University on June 15, 1920. From 1920–21, she served as a house medical officer of the Johns Hopkins Hospital and as assistant resident in psychiatry from 1922–25. During the years 1923–25, Dr. Thompson also held an appointment as Instructor in Psychiatry in conjunction with her staff appointment.

As for courses in psychoanalysis during the years 1916–25, I have been unable to find any mention of specific courses in the catalogues for those years. Perhaps special lectures were given; however, they are not described. Unfortunately, there is no one presently in the Department of Psychiatry who was on the resident staff or faculty at that time to supply the information you desire.

Herbert Spencer Jennings, who was on the faculty of the Johns Hopkins University from 1906–1947, never held a faculty appointment in the School of Medicine. He might well have lectured in the medical school; however, there is no record of such teaching.

Sincerely,

Mary E. Burke, Registrar

I hope that in telling Clara Mabel Thompson's story, I have added to what is known, and hopefully made it a little more accurate. As in the oral history tradition I encourage others to keep the story alive.

References

Burke, M. (1961). [Letter to Maurice Green]. The Alan Mason Chesney Medical Archives, The Johns Hopkins University, The Johns Hopkins Hospital.

Capelle, E. (1998). Clara Thompson as culturalist. *Psychoanalytic Review, 85* (1), 75–93.

Capelle, E. L. (1993). *Analyzing the "modern woman": Psychoanalytic debates about feminism, 1920–1950* [Unpublished doctoral dissertation, Columbia University].

D'Ercole, A. (1999). Designing the lesbian subject: Looking backwards, looking forwards. In R. Lesser & E. Schoenberg (Eds.), *That obscure subject of desire: An interdisciplinary study of Freud's female homosexual.* pp. 115–129 Routledge.

D'Ercole, A. (2012). Nella mia famiglia: Race, gender and the intergenerational dilemmas of being a witness. *Contemporary Psychoanalysis, 48*(4), 451–482.

D'Ercole, A., & Struening, E. (1990). Victimization among homeless women: Implications for service delivery. *Journal of Community Psychology, 18*(2), 141–152.

D'Ercole, A., & Waxenberg, B. (1999). Beyond the feminine ideal: The body speaks. In M. Dimen & A. Harris (Eds.), *Storms in her head.* pp. 303–322 Other Press.

Dupont, J. (Ed.). (1988). *The clinical diary of Sándor Ferenczi.* Harvard University Press.

Falzeder, E. (2015). *Psychoanalytic filiations: Mapping the psychoanalytic movement.* Karnac Books.

Freud, S. (1952a). *Interview with Clara Thompson (K. R. Eissler, Interviewer).* Manuscript/Mixed Material. Sigmund Freud Papers: Interviews and Recollections, Set A, 1914–1998 (Box 122). Manuscripts Division, Library of Congress, Washington, DC. www.loc.gov/item/mss3999001575/

Green, M. (1961). Letter to Registrar at Johns Hopkins Medical School. Alan Mason Chesney Medical Archives of Johns Hopkins Medicine, Nursing, and Public Health.

Green, M. (Ed.). (1964a). Her life. In M. Green (Ed.), *Interpersonal psychoanalysis: The selected papers of Clara M. Thompson.* Basic Books pp. 347–377.

Green, M. (Ed.). (1964b). *Interpersonal psychoanalysis: The selected papers of Clara M. Thompson.* Basic Books.

Menaker, E. (1989). *Appointment in Vienna: An American psychoanalyst recalls her student days in pre-war Austria.* St. Martin's.

Milburn, N., & D'Ercole, A. (Eds.). (1991a). Homeless women, children and families. *The American Psychologist, 46*(11), 1159–1160.

Milburn, N., & D'Ercole, A. (1991b). Homeless women: Moving towards a comprehensive model. *The American Psychologist, 46*(11), 1161–1169.

Thompson, C. (1938). Notes on the psychoanalytic significance of choice of analyst. *Psychiatry, 1*(2), pp. 205–216.

Chapter 1

Interview With Dr. Clara Thompson

Sigmund Freud Papers:
Speaking Her Mind

Background of the Interview

Beginning the story of Clara Thompson's life and work with this historically important interview presents two distinct and rare opportunities. It is
an occasion to hear directly from Clara Thompson about her experiences
and it also lays out the framework for an understanding of Thompson's
role in the history of psychoanalysis. By the time of this June 4, 1952,
interview, Thompson's position within psychoanalysis has been firmly
established. She is 58 years old, a trailblazing founder of interpersonal
psychoanalysis, the foundational and theoretical home of relational psychoanalysis, and a founder and Director of the William Alanson White
Institute of Psychiatry, Psychoanalysis, and Psychology. Dr. Kurt Eissler,
her interviewer, is the creator and Director of the Sigmund Freud Archives.
He has collected thousands of tapes, letters, papers, and interviews for the
archive and arranged for them to be held in the Library of Congress.

Thompson and Eissler are representatives of opposing factions in battles that include disputes about psychoanalytic techniques and metapsy-
chology; issues of regulation and power; and the essence of the aim of
psychoanalysis itself. They emerged from these years of controversy with
dissimilar reputations: Thompson as a leader of a non-Freudian movement, Interpersonal Psychoanalysis; Eissler, as a confidant of Anna Freud,
"the pope" of orthodox Freudian psychoanalysis (Malcolm, 2000).

The interview sets the stage for an understanding and appreciation of
Clara Thompson's role in the development of psychoanalysis during a
period in its history when significant changes in techniques were formulated. It follows the time when Thompson was in psychoanalytic treatment
with Sándor Ferenczi in Budapest as he was formulating his innovative theories, and when she was his collaborator. Together Ferenczi and Thompson

DOI: 10.4324/9781003261797-2

were breaking from Freud and establishing a new philosophy and technique that is foundational to interpersonal/relational psychoanalysis. Her role was both as an observer and participant. Not only was she in "the room where it happened," she caused things to happen. One could easily designate her the leader of the American Interpersonal Psychoanalytic tradition. In fact, Green (1964) did just that when he coined the term "Interpersonal Psycho-analysis" as the title of the book he edited of her collected papers. Thompson, however, might have frowned on any notion that she was an anointed leader, because she would disapprove of her name being linked with any "movement" or group that suggested orthodoxy or rigid conventions.

Thompson's close friend and colleague—and her third analyst—Erich Fromm (see *Clara M. Thompson's Professional Evolution and Legacy: An American Psychoanalyst (1933–1958)*) claimed that her personal characteristics complemented the demands of the newly developing disciple of psychoanalysis (Fromm, 1964). Fromm's tribute, published in part as the *Foreword* to her collected papers, portrays her as a woman who "acted according to her own convictions." She stood by her friends, and was loyal, never intimidating . . . nor could she be intimidated. She had "integrity" which "made it possible for others to trust her and rely on her. She had an appreciation for theory, but she also had "common sense." All this while remaining a "warm, devoted, and nurturant person" (p. vi).

Fromm's tribute to Thompson highlights the positive aspects of her life and elicits an emotional connection. The memorial tribute to Kurt Eissler by the *New Yorker* writer Janet Malcolm (2000) is also positive and reveals parts of Eissler's persona:

> Encountering Eissler at a gathering of analysts was like coming upon an orchid in a hayfield. Coupled with his erudition, subtlety of mind and exquisite (perhaps mildly ironic) courtesy was a bracing, sometimes almost abrasive, honesty. He was thorny and passionate. He always spoke his mind. There was nothing smooth and glossy about him. Like all people of superior achievement, he was too intelligent to be satisfied, no less impressed with himself. He revered genius but did not disdain lesser minds, never appearing to notice the disparity between himself and even the most dull-witted of his interlocutors. His extraordinary kindness was well known, not because he ever spoke of it, but because there were so many beneficiaries of it.
>
> (p. 33)

Malcolm seems genuinely affected by accounts of Eissler's sharp intelligence and the style of his personal presentation.

> Eissler had always guarded his privacy; little more was known about his personal life than that he was married to another distinguished analyst, Ruth Eissler, and that he took his analyst's August vacation in Vinalhaven, ME. He and his wife were childless, and he was given to forming fatherly friendships with younger men and women. His final decades were shadowed by the unwelcome publicity that one of these friendships brought down on him. To the world at large, Eissler is known only as the guileless analyst who was betrayed and sued by his protege Jeffrey Masson.
>
> (p. 33)

Psychoanalysis and its practices were the center of both Thompson and Eissler's lives. However, Thompson left a coterie of colleagues and students who utter her name with affection. Eissler's name is publicly associated with Jeffrey Masson (1985) and the scandal that erupted in the 1980s around Freud's seduction theory (Rachman, 2018).

By the time of this interview, Clara Thompson had a lifelong dedication to developing a treatment process that is distinctively caring, authentic, and democratic and creating a psychoanalytic training program accessible to both medical and non-medical professionals. She was a leader with experience across a broad range of organizational issues. She warned her students that psychoanalytic institutes can have all the satisfactions and evils of a family, stimulating dependencies and rivalries that can hamper their independent development (Thompson, 1958).

We meet this pioneering woman for the first time in this interview as a thoroughly independent person, averse to bureaucratic power structures yet firmly embedded within them.

In this conversation, Thompson's voice comes across as amiable and forthcoming, while Eissler is both collegial, warm, and restrained. At times, the reader can feel puzzled, especially if expecting an interview that is modeled after a detailed inquiry or listening with the proverbial third ear to what is not being said. It would have been helpful to see their body language, feel the atmosphere, and experience the tone of the dialogue. As Stern (2019) wisely advises, meaningfulness is "more than just words" (p. 1).

Yet, this is the Clara Thompson we want to get to know, to understand. She is at the top of her game, and she is speaking to a professional opponent for posterity since she is aware that what she says will be preserved within the Freud Archives.

The interview most probably occurred at Eissler's office in the Olmstead, a Beaux-Arts building at 285 Central Park West. It is an iconic building that features large windows and views that float above Central Park. Nellie Thompson, Curator of Archives at New York Psychoanalytic Institute, found a letter dated July 1, 1952, addressed to Eissler at 285 CPW. She, therefore, surmises "that it would seem to be the address where the Thompson interview took place" (personal communication, September 30, 2019). Eissler lived at The El Dorado at 300 Central Park West a few doors down from his office. Thompson was living across the park on the upper east side.

Thompson and Eissler were interested in Freud and Ferenczi and in the relationship between them. The Freud and Ferenczi correspondence (Falzeder et al., 2000) gives evidence of how Freud, as the founder of psychoanalysis, and Ferenczi, as his favorite disciple, helped shape psychoanalysis for more than two decades.

Thompson's Relationship With Ferenczi

Unlike Thompson, Ferenczi grew up surrounded by volumes of political writings in his father's bookstore. That world was lost to him when his "free thinking" father died, leaving the young Ferenczi bereft at age fifteen (Rachman, 2018). Between 1908 and 1919, Freud (age 52) and Ferenczi (age 35) found each other and for a time were inseparable. Ferenczi discovered in Freud the lost father of ideas, where Freud found an accomplished and devoted son. By 1926, after Ferenczi gave a series of lectures on psychoanalysis in New York, their relationship began to deteriorate (Falzeder et al., 2000). Freud became increasingly critical of Ferenczi for his clinical innovations. In 1932, Ferenczi read his paper, "Confusion of Tongues Between Adults and the Child: The Language of Tenderness and Passion," to Freud. According to Thompson, Freud was disturbed by the paper and did not want him to publish it. More devastating for Ferenczi was that when he extended his hand to Freud at the end of the visit, Freud turned away. Freud thought Ferenczi was heading down a wrong path, one that would return psychoanalysis to the seduction theory. Clara Thompson was in psychoanalysis with Ferenczi during this period. It is a time when both men were plagued by illnesses, which could have strengthened their growing differences (Falzeder et al., 2000) resulting in their relationship becoming attenuated and distant (Rachman, 1997).

In this interview (courtesy of Dr. Emanuel E. Garcia, the literary executor of the K.R. Eissler Estate) Thompson dates the disturbance in the Freud–Ferenczi relationship to a time prior to the "Confusion of Tongues"[1] paper, a time before she started her treatment with Ferenczi.

The Interview[2]
   Clara Thompson, M.D. Interviewed by K. R. Eissler, M.D.
June 4, 1952.

DR. E.: Will you be kind enough to tell me xxxxx ^whatever you can tell me about Ferenczi, particularly in his connection with Professor Freud?

DR. T.: Well, I know much more about Ferenczi then I do about Freud, after all. When I first went to Buda Pest in 1928, I expected to visit Freud also on my way there or going home, and Ferenczi didn't want me to go and meet Freud. And this was the first that I had any inkling that they were not on friendly terms. He told me that Freud did not like to meet women any more because of his mouth; but since then I knew many women who did meet him, so I think maybe that was not quite the fact. But of course I had just begun analysis so he didn't tell me anything/^very specific at that time. I know when Ferenczi came to America he was very eager to introduce lay analysis here, and he came with all the enthusiasm of ~~freeih~~ ^bringing word from Freud.

DR. E.: Ferenczi?

DR. T.: Yes.

DR. E.: In what year was that?

                                                          (Freud, 1952a, p. 1)

Let's pause here to think about what just transpired. Thompson believed Ferenczi kept her from Freud for reasons other than what he said. She gives Eissler the opening for more probing questions, but he seems to avert his attention from what Thompson has disclosed. The next question Eissler reaches for is, "What year was that?"

Eissler is more interested in trying to pinpoint the beginning of the tension between Freud and Ferenczi than learning more about Thompson's experience. For her part, Thompson could easily have added her views as to why Ferenczi misled her, but she elects to not go down that path. To complicate the picture, Thompson was aware (see comments later in the interview) that Elizabeth Severn[3] wished to visit Freud and that Ferenczi provided a letter of introduction for her in 1925 (Freud, 1952b). The question of Thompson's interest in meeting Freud appears and reappears in this interview. It could be that Ferenczi was by 1927 feeling the tension in his relationship with Freud and in a protective move kept her from meeting with Freud.

Why ask, "What year was that?" The year may be important in that it might mark the time when Freud became angry with Ferenczi, but it's hard to know for certain. We know Ferenczi was on friendly terms with Freud when he published his elasticity paper in 1928 (Rachman, 1997). Ferenczi was still on good terms when he came to America to promote Freud and lay analysis but American analysts were very critical of non-medically trained analysts, so he received a cool welcome.

With the introduction of lay analysis, Thompson has brought a key controversy of the early years of psychoanalysis in America into the conversation. The issue of training "lay analysts" goes to the heart of a dispute that divided American psychoanalysts for decades. Eisold (2018) explains that to establish their claim to psychoanalysis, American psychiatrists felt they had to police their profession to keep out entrepreneurs or what was perceived as "ill trained 'quacks'" (p. 38). That included all non-physicians. They argued that failing to do this would lead to a lack of professional authority needed from both their patients and their medical colleagues.

Over the years, this disagreement disrupted and stirred up disputes in many analytic organizations, and Thompson was intimately involved in all these struggles. With that history as background, it is striking that of all the questions Eissler might have asked, he chooses "in what year was that?" And Thompson answers his question with her own concrete answer:

DR. T.: That was in 1926, I think, when he taught at The New School. And he met with a great deal of hostility, and I think he was very unhappy here, because all the analysts were very much against this and he therefore felt sort of left out. Well, that's for that. (Freud, 1952a, p. 1)

We are not certain what she means when she says, "Well, that's for that." The idiom can denote the end of the discussion, or it can connote "that's that" (i.e., the matter is settled). It is unclear which of these Thompson is claiming. With the risk of being accused of analyzing Thompson, it's hard not to imagine that she is signaling to Eissler that she still harbors strong feelings about that experience. She undoubtedly felt left out by Ferenczi's move to keep her from Freud. She was aware that other people in Ferenczi's practice were introduced to Freud, for example, Elizabeth Severn, who had met with Freud twice. Some of her colleagues had not only met Freud but were in treatment with him. Specifically, Thompson's friend from medical school, Edith Jackson, was a patient of Freud's while she was in treatment with Ferenczi. The foursome—Freud, Jackson, Ferenczi, and Thompson— form a significant web of interrelationships in psychoanalytic history. Their rivalry and competitiveness led to some acting out of feelings referred to as the famous "kissing episode" (see Chapter 4). Another question that begins to form from this exchange is the question of why Thompson didn't override Ferenczi and approach Freud herself? Thompson cont'd:

Then, I went—you see I was analyzed in chunks by Ferenczi. I went there first in 1928 for two months, then I went in 1929 for two months, then I went in 1930 for three months, and then I was there from '31 to '33. And by 1930 I think the situation was much more tense between him and Freud. I didn't hear much about it in 1929; he seemed to be very popular still in the International. I went to the Oxford Congress, and he was there. I mean not Freud, but Ferenczi, and everything seemed to be going very well. In 1930 I didn't hear very much either, but after I started, stayed, with him for two years he, it became more and more an issue, and he was already having difficulties in publishing what he wrote, with the feeling that Freud advised him very strongly against this. At that time, of course, he was very much in the grips of his theory of the relaxation technique, which Freud felt was very dangerous. He told me that, that Freud felt it was very dangerous, and that he thought it was very dangerous to give patients love, that it was very dangerous to encourage them to relive so actively as Ferenczi did. Also, another innovation of Ferenczi's at that time disturbed Freud a lot, and that was having the patient, telling the patients your faults—telling the patient what was wrong with you.

(Freud, 1952a, pp. 1–2)

Thompson recounts the essence of Ferenczi's new therapeutic techniques and Freud's reaction to them. The number of times she uses the word "dangerous" should sound an alarm, but Eissler does not seem disturbed; he replies with "Yes." His yes is like a Freudian nod, a signal to continue—and Thompson does:

DR. E.: Yes.

DR. T.: That is not in the sense of giving, of letting him analyze you—although he did have a patient who did that, too,—I am sure—but, rather, that if the patient knew correctly what was going on, or if he guessed that you were angry, or something like that, it would be better to tell the patient, because otherwise you were repeating the childhood picture of the authoritarian father. I know that a friend of mine was being analyzed by Freud at that time—Edith Jackson, I suppose you know her?

DR. E.: Yes.

DR. T.: And she said she talked about this to Anna Freud, and Anna Freud came to feel that this was quite a dangerous thing, to, to do, to admit that you have faults to the patient. Oh, I mean I don't know what Anna Freud said, xxxx because I didn't have the contact myself. Then Freud began writing his letters, which seemed to be in the nature of scolding him, as far as I could make out. Ferenczi translated parts of them to me. (Did anybody by chance get in touch with his step-daughter?)

DR. E.: No, not yet. The correspondence is preserved, it is in London, but I have not yet contacted her.

DR. T.: So, I—he translated it to me, pieces of it, and I know that, well what I told you in the letter, the chief thing that I remember is just that: that he told him he was in his second childhood and that he was trying to make up to patients for the love he needed, and that he was trying to get from patients the love he needed. And I think there probably was some truth in that, except that it wasn't useful to Ferenczi to be told that as a scolding parent being horrified at what his child was doing. Another thing that Ferenczi always felt very unhappy about was that he couldn't get more analysis with Freud—or with any one, for that matter. I don't know why. He probably couldn't go to anybody but Freud, in his own mind. He apparently felt very strongly the need of more analysis all his life, and I think that towards the end that he did really use his patients in order to try to solve his own problems.

(Freud, 1952a, pp. 2–3)

This is a highly significant thing for Thompson to say for a few reasons. Thompson disagreed with Ferenczi's thoughts about love.

DR. T:

I mean that he would do more than just say, "Yes, I felt this way." He would tell—I know towards the, his last illness he told me a great deal about his early life and about his unhappiness, about his sexual escapades and things like that. I think by that time he was already mentally quite disturbed. That was in the last winter, 1932, or 33, 1932 or 33.

DR. E.: His sickness affected him that much? It was pernicious anemia, no?

(Freud, 1952a, p. 3)

Thompson confirms that Ferenczi was mentally affected by his anemia, but a far cry from Jones's (1953) destructive allegation that Ferenczi was mentally disturbed in the last years of his life. It was Ernest Jones who describes Ferenczi's last contributions to psychoanalysis as tainted by a mental deterioration based on a progressive psychosis (Bonomi, 1999).

Bonomi (1999) examined historical documents and found that they did not support Jones's allegations. On the other hand, Bonomi surmises that Jones's accusation was part of a conspiracy, not "a one-man fabrication," because the analytic community was trying to discredit Ferenczi's therapeutic experiments with Freud's method by taking aim at his general emotional instability. Thompson's and Fromm's responses to those false charges are discussed later.

DR. T.: I think it was pernicious anemia.[4] I know he had a red count of about a million and a half when he fell in the railroad station, and that they had great difficulty in treating him because he already had a kidney condition and wouldn't take massive doses of liver.[5] His mind was definitely affected, I can tell you that. He had combined sclerosis symptoms, I mean he staggered and he was not sure of his walking.

Now, Ferenczi always had a great awkwardness of his hands. I don't know if you ever noticed it. So that how much of that was sort of constitutional, I don't know, but he certainly got to the point where he was not sure of his walking. He also—the time when I finally realized that he must be very mentally disturbed was one morning he didn't come in. I was his first patient, and I was waiting in the waiting room, and he didn't come in until finally somebody told him I was there—it was, oh, half an hour after the time—and he didn't seem to be at all concerned that he had overlooked it. There was a very great smoothness to his attitude. And that morning I noticed that his face was very red, and I said, "have you been sitting in the sun?" And he said, "No, no." And I said that he looked, that his face looked red and he brushed that off, too, and didn't want to know anything about that. Also his wife told me that during his last illness he was xxx ^{often} reading the paper up-side-down, just sitting holding it. And I think there were other evidences of memory disturbances, so that his mind must have been quite affected. I think that Freud tried to make out that possibly that was why some of his behavior was what Freud considered so extreme in his treatment of patients. I unfortunately am in a way involved in the struggle with Freud because I was talking with Edith Jackson about his new technique, and she said, "You mean that you actually kiss Ferenczi?" And I said, "Sure, I kiss him any time I want to," And she of course at once went back and told this to Freud and Freud became very upset about this and wrote him quite a letter about it. I must say that Ferenczi was very decent to me. He was very upset, naturally, and, you see I had proceeded on the theory well if this is what we do, why don't we admit it? and he finally admitted that I was right, that if he was going to do such things, he should admit them and not try to hide it from Freud. Ferenczi was very afraid of Freud all his life. He felt that Freud despised people, and he would give examples such as this:/ ^{He said} One day he was talking about these "swine of patients"—Freud was—and then he said one day he was talking about a homosexual and he spit on the ground as he talked about him.

(Freud, 1952a, pp. 3–4)

I don't think we have heard this line repeated before in any discussion of Freud's attitude toward same-sex sexualities. It offends still to hear it here. Thompson goes on to talk about Ferenczi:

Thompson cont'd

I think, as you know, Ferenczi was very sympathetic to homosexuals. I don't know whether he ever was homosexual as a young man or not. There were certain qualities in him that makes me think he might have had some strong tendencies that way, and as you know he married very late—near 50, I guess, when he married. However, he lived for many years with her before that and she was married to somebody else. He became more and more bitter about the Freud authoritarian attitude but he, unlike the other rebels, was unable to break with him, he was unable to establish himself separately. He was always, as you know from his writings, trying to appease Freud, trying to say, "It's really not anything different from what you've already said. I'm just making it a little bit more intense." But it was he, I think, who made me feel that Freud—that there quite a difference in the attitude toward patients of these two men, that that Freud was more—contemptuous is too strong a word, but—less interested in them as people, and Ferenczi had a very strong positive feeling towards the patient, which I think was not necessarily, it was not bad—not even necessarily—was not bad, that his real respect for sick people was very great.

(Freud, 1952a, p. 4)

Thompson has disclosed a great deal in this paragraph. First, and significantly, she alludes to Freud's disparagement of homosexuality. This attitude has a long and deep history that has been chronicled by Drescher (1996, 1997, 2008). In tracing the evolving attitudes toward homosexuality within organized psychoanalysis, Drescher situates Freud's views on the topic within a historical context. We owe Drescher a debt of gratitude for his sustained and unrelenting work to reveal the discriminatory and harmful practices within psychoanalysis. He suggests that Freud, for his time, had a more tolerant attitude, quoting Freud's (1935) now-famous Letter to an American Mother:

Homosexuality is assuredly no advantage, but it is nothing to be ashamed of, no vice, no degradation; it cannot be classified as an illness; we consider it to be a variation of the sexual function, produced by a certain arrest of sexual development . . . By asking me if I can help, you mean, I suppose, if I can abolish homosexuality and make normal heterosexuality take its place. The answer is, in a general way, we cannot promise to achieve it. In a certain number of cases we succeed in developing the blighted germs of heterosexual tendencies, which are present in every homosexual, in the majority of cases it is no more possible.

(Freud, 1935, pp. 423–424)

This is an older and wiser Freud than the earlier one who displayed derision. Perhaps his attitude was tempered under the influence of Ferenczi, who held a more moderate attitude toward homosexuality. Freud did sign a 1930 petition to decriminalize homosexuality and, Ferenczi, in the early 1900s, offered his patient Rosa K., a frequently arrested transsexual, a letter for her to give to police that said she should not be arrested because she had what was considered at the time to be a mental disorder. Rachman (1997) points out that both Ferenczi and Winnicott were the target of homophobic gossip, because they introduced maternal relationships into the analytic discourse and because they were more empathic and tender in their approach to patients. Both tenderness and empathy were viewed as "female" characteristics.

Drescher (2008) argues that although Freud "did not consider homosexuality an illness, his theory did not quite constitute a clean bill of health— calling someone immature, rather than sick, is not as offensive, but neither appellation is particularly respectful" (p. 446). Second, Thompson reveals her own shades of prejudice in her speculation that Ferenczi's late marriage was a potential indication of his homosexuality. In her analysis and in her own writings, we never hear her use this criterion to make this connection between her sexuality and the fact that she never married or that she too found a partner late in life. Thompson's own bisexuality is scarcely mentioned except by Zeborah Schachtel,[6] who in my interview with her described Thompson as "bi-sexual" (personal communication, May 2016).

In Thompson's (1947) essay "Changing Concepts of Homosexuality in Psychoanalysis," she argues there are different cultural attitudes toward gender non-conforming boys and girls, with less tolerance for boys' atypical behavior than girls'. She also makes progressive statements in that essay about same-sex couples and the viability of their marriages. Of course, by the time of Eissler's interview, the deep conventionalism of the mid-20th century had set in:

American culture vigorously persecuted homosexuality from the 1940s through the 1960s, at a time when the theories of analysts like

Rado, Bieber, and Socarides predominated in psychoanalytic organizations. Not surprisingly, in those years, patients and analysts usually began treatment with a shared view that homosexuality was a problem requiring treatment.

(Drescher, 2008, p. 454)

Thompson had already reviewed Bergler's works (1939, 1940, 1956), which held strong anti-homosexual attitudes. Was she influenced by these prejudicial ideas? Given Thompson's deep sense of independence, it is hard to think that her ideas were influenced by the then current *zeitgeist*, but there may be an unexamined blind spot in her that we are up against. In any case, Eissler does not follow up on any of these comments.

DR. E.: Did he tell you something about his own analysis with Freud?

DR. T.: No.

DR. E.: of Freud's technique?

DR. T.: No, he never told me much about that. He as I said,[he said]: "I only had six months and I needed more, and he told me I could get along with that." I think perhaps the fact that he was so far away from Vienna made it possible for him to keep more of an illusion and fight less directly with Freud.

DR. E.: He spoke English with you, or?

DR. T.: Yes, he spoke English.

DR. E.: He spoke English well?

DR. T.: No. He spoke it adequately but not well. I mean he had a very large vocabulary, but he had a very bad Hungarian accent and he had great difficulty with the grammar, but you could always manage to find out what he was talking about.

DR. E.: You didn't learn Hungarian?

DR. T.: Oh, I learned quite a few words. I lived there two years, you see. I learned to get around the city with taxi men and in restaurants—such words, words you use in everyday life, but otherwise I didn't learn the language.

DR. E.: Did he tell you something about how he got in analysis, how his interest in analysis was provoked?

DR. T.: No, I don't think he—I think I got what little I know of that from reading his notes, those that were published recently in the International Journal. I never knew those things about it.

DR. E.: And didn't he speak about the early days of psychoanalysis and its development?

DR. T.: He spoke about the Salzburg Congress, and about how, what a naïve man he had been, that he had thought, "Now, here is a bunch of psychoanalysts. They're all trying to be honest with themselves. We will all get together and we'll talk about our problems and we'll help each other." And he said, "Wasn't that naïve?" And apparently he became aware that the tremendous competition that went on among those practically unanalyzed people was very great. I think he always fantasied himself as Freud's favorite son, in some way. Not in the way of strength, I somehow—I don't know how to say it clearly, it seems to me but/ it seems to me his dependency on Freud was that of a very loving son, and very, very dependent on him. And, yet, I w also feel that he struggled his whole life to reconcile his own thinking with Freud's, which didn't go, and that's why one gets the impression from his writings that such extreme conformity with Freud—I think you can't read his work without xxxx realizing that immediately he talks about patients, whereas Freud talks about theory. Immediately he brings/ in in the examples of people a living type of thing. But, well, what he told me about his change from his deprivation technique—you know, this extreme one—into what he later called his relaxation technique, therapy, was that he felt that he had never really believed in the deprivation idea, and that he thought that some devil in him had forced him to carry it to such extremes that it would prove it was absurd. And of course his shift to the relaxation therapy was largely due to Elisabeth La Verne who was his patient. I would say she was a paranoid bitch.

DR. E.: I know nothing about that.

DR. T.: This shouldn't be published, should it? But she was one of those very controlling, hypochondriacal women, extreme hypochondriacal types. You know the kind that would have to have emergency operations and nothing be solved (?) and so forth. And she could never get up. She spent most of her life in bed, where she ruled from her bed.

(Freud, 1952a, pp. 4–6)

For Thompson, the stalwart New Englander, taking to one's bed might have bordered on the obscene. Yet Thompson gives Severn the credit she deserves for her inspiring collaboration with Ferenczi (Rachman, 2018), and she offers it despite holding her own negative and aggressively expressed opinion of Severn as "a paranoid bitch." Eissler does not react to this information.

Thompson cont'd

She had her daughter under her thumb, and so forth, and she presently had Ferenczi, and I think the last three, the last two years when I was there, there was quite a change in him, and I think he was quite under her influence and that it was she who demanded the endless hours. You know it started his idea that maybe, one hour a day isn't enough; if the patient needs more, you should give it to him. And I think that much of this was his attempt to solve the problems of this woman.

DR. E.: What happened to her later, do you know?

DR. T.: She's practicing here in New York City.

DR. E.: She's an analyst?

DR. T.: She's a lay analyst, yes. In fact she lives about five blocks from here, I think.

DR. E.: And she lost her hypochondriasis?

DR. T.: No. I don't think so. She left Ferenczi about three months before he died. He finally got the strength to dismiss her, and the day he did, he went into a kind of an elation. Her parting words to him were that he would die, that she would see that he died, and that he would be a little man and completely forgotten by the world. This was her parting curse. She was the sort of person who was psychic. She really had a lot of extrasensory perception, although a lot of it, too, I think was fake with her. I mean I think she was quite a show-off. But one thing xxx that startled me about Ferenczi early in my treatment was she sug —he suggested would I like to live with her, she had a villa, she had rented a villa and she wanted somebody to live with her. So I went up to see her and she started to tell me, well, now I mustn't make a noise at such hours and I must use this room and I must not use that room, and that when she had certain people I must go out of the house. Well, so I said, no, I didn't want the thing. And Ferenczi suddenly said, "Why, you had courage." And, it had never occurred to me that this was an emotionally tinged situation until then. I thought if somebody offers you a room and you don't take the terms, they aren't suitable, and so you say no. But apparently he would have been afraid to say no to her, in that situation. I used to call her "Bird of prey". She looked like one. Oh, she told me—why did I get off on her? She told me that she was the greatest analyst in the world because she had no hate. Well, she was remarkable.

DR. E.: I can imagine.

DR. T.: It's difficult to imagine because it's stuck out all over her. But she had no hate as long as she could control people. But her parting curse shows how much love she had. Of course he was then seriously ill. That was in February; he died in May. So she probably thought it was a good curse, it probably would work. I saw him about three days before he died.

DR. E.: He was still working?

DR. T.: No, he stopped working about the first of May and he died I think the twenty-third of May. But I stayed around there, I don't know why, I just stayed. I had some patients with me and I'd planned to stay, so I stayed. I didn't see any point in going home somehow; it seemed—I don't think we quite faced the fact that he was dying. I don't know why we didn't, except I don't seem ever to face that fact about people.

(Freud, 1952a, pp. 6–8)

The sorrow in Thompson's words does not appear to reach Eissler. She moves from discussing Elizabeth Severn's character and her burden on Ferenczi to her own sadness and her reliance on denial in the face of Ferenczi's death—and death in general. By the time of this interview, Thompson has lost many loved ones, including her father, her mother (in the year of the interview), Sullivan, and her soul mate, Henry Major.

DR. E.: And do you remember that last meeting?

DR. T.: Yes, because he was in bed and I went in and was talking with him and he kept saying goodby to me in indirect ways, and I, several times I said, "But I'm coming to see you again this week," and then he'd say, "Oh, yes," and then again he would say goodby and he'd tell me what I should do in America, that I should carry on his ideas, and so forth. And I'd say, "but I'm not leaving Budapest, I'm coming to see you in a few days," and he'd say, "Oh, yes," but I think he must have felt that he would never see me again. He had a great many phobias I gather from what I've heard. A great deal of physical anxiety about his health all his life.

DR. E.: Yes?

DR. T.: So this Mrs. La Verne told me. She said—I don't know how authentic anything she said is—but she said he used to tie his tongue with a string every night so he wouldn't swallow it. Tie it to the bed, or something like that. It sounds too fantastic.

DR. E.: Yes.

DR. T.: Well, I doubt that, but, I think he was, really—because he did ask me to look at his pupils to see if he really had Argyle Robertson pupils. Apparently he had some theory he had paresis[7] (?). Well, he didn't have Argyle Robertson pupils, so I'd tell him that, tell him the truth about that. And then one of the last times, I think pretty nearly the last analytic hour I had with him, he suddenly took me into the next room and played a Victrola record of—I don't remember what it was, but it was about somebody longing for love—and he wept over this record. And, this, he just played it as something which—well, it was something I was talking about. He was completely in it, too.

DR. E.: What made him feel so alone?

DR. T.: I think that it must have been his neurosis. I think that he was the middle son of a very large family. I think that he was one of these people who had a neurotic need for love, who counted on this as a way of feeling secure; and I think that's why he was so ingratiating, so—such a sweet person—where he played always to get affection. I think he was also quite impressed with status. But I guess most Europeans have that more than Americans do.

DR. E.: Yes.

DR. T.: It was always a surprise to me because it didn't seem to me to go with the rest of his character, somehow.

DR. E.: In what way did that show up?

DR. T.: Well, he—there was a man that was being analyzed by him, Teddy Miller, who was just an ordinary lower East Side Jew, a Polish Jew, who, with no education at all but plenty of money, and I know that he was very friendly to most of the Americans who were with him—at least he would see us once in a while socially, but he would never invite him until the very end, and he told me once that he was ashamed of him. He was ashamed to have him in his house. And the man wasn't so crude as all that. I think that it was, there was some worship, of intellect—not intellect, education, culture, that he couldn't overcome. And I think he was also very much impressed that there, say with Alice Lowell, for instance, because of her American aristocratic background. And

DR. E.: Alice Lowell?

DR. T.: Yes. She was also a patient when I was. And I think he was rather ashamed of me. Now this may be a patient's projection, but I also was a person whom he almost never invited to his house. Although his wife told me after he died that he had often told her I would be his best pupil, that he felt I would be his best pupil. Now, I, well I believe he must have said that, but somehow he was not—I didn't have enough polish to, to make him comfortable.

(Freud, 1952a, pp. 8–9)

Are we hearing now why Ferenczi had kept Thompson away from Freud? Was Ferenczi so concerned with how he was seen (by Freud) that he didn't want Freud to think that his best pupil was someone without "enough polish"? Is this really about Clara Thompson?

Thompson had an outstanding American education, including medical school, and was upwardly mobile in the American sense of going beyond her parents in professional status. But she was an American with different customs and values, and Ferenczi may have been a bit of a snob; Thompson, for her part, may have felt intimidated and not a part of the European culture. Her comment to her friend Schachtel (personal communication, May 2016) that she did not consider herself an intellectual, when she was an accomplished scholar, suggests a lack of confidence but if anything, Thompson was consistently modest. In "Ferenczi's Contributions to Psychoanalysis" (1944), she clearly states, "Ferenczi was Hungarian . . . he tended to be overly impressed by status . . . He preferred his sentimental tendencies and struggled against his conventional trends" (p. 45).

Thompson may have been silently comparing herself to other American patients of Ferenczi including, her friend Alice Lowell, an upper-class descendant of the famous Lowells of Massachusetts (Sankovitch, 2017). Ferenczi openly admired Alice Lowell, which could have set up some sibling-like competition. Could Thompson have had an intimate relationship with Alice Lowell or Izette de Forest, each bisexual, and all three New Englanders and simultaneous patients of Ferenczi (see Chapter 5)? So far there is only confirmation regarding Lowell and de Forest.

DR. E.: Why did he discontinue analysis? I mean why was it—you said first two months, then—

DR. T.: That was because of money. I mean, well I was just a young analyst here in Baltimore, and I had—well, I managed to save say a Thou-
sand Dollars one year so I could go over for two months; and then the
next year I saved that much more; and then when I finally went for two
years, I took eight patients with me, and in that way I was able to stay
there. I had no money except what I earned. I had no background of
money at all. So,

(Freud, 1952a, pp. 9–10)

It was common for a certain educated class of Americans to travel to
Europe, and even more so for psychiatrists and others interested in psy-
choanalysis. There were very few analysts in the United States at that time
(Menaker, 1989).

DR. E.: Did he ever tell you why he didn't want you to go to see Freud?
DR. T.: He never told me except when he told me the first time.
DR. E.: He never told—
DR. T.: I never took it up with him again, but it became more and more
apparent that he was xxxxxxxx uncomfortable to have his pupils meet
Freud; but I also wanted to call on Helene Deutsch at that time, and
he didn't want me to go to see her. But that he said was because he
didn't like her.
DR. E.: Did he tell you why he didn't like her?
DR. T.: He said he thought she was a hypocrite. He felt that she was a—
that she didn't tell the truth in her papers.

(Freud, 1952a, p. 10)

Thompson tosses this line out like a hand grenade—Helene Deutsch[8] was
a hypocrite and she didn't tell the truth in her papers! But Eissler is undis-
turbed and switches the topic. And yet, an interesting side note is that
Esther Menaker[9] didn't like Deutsch either. She described her as a "rigid
and relentlessly critical psychoanalyst" (Menaker, 1989, p. 55).

DR. E.: How did you happen to go ^ to Ferenczi?
DR. T.: I was—I met him when he was here at The New School, and he
was the first analyst I had ever seen I thought I could talk to. I don't
think I could have been analyzed any more in an ᵃ more authoritarian way
at that time any way. xxx One can stand anything now, I guess. I would

find it very difficult. I also have a very great need of love, which I think I couldn't have stood the deprivation in orthodox analysis.

DR. E.: And you made arrangements with Ferenczi when he was here in—

DR. T.: When he was here I wanted to come to him, when he was here, but his time was all filled and he said, "Well, why don't you come to Budapest?" And I said, "Well, how can I? I can't afford it." And he said, "Well, couldn't you save money and come?" And he said, "How long would it take you to save money?" And I said, "Well, maybe two years." He said, "All right, let's make it in two years." Well, then I forgot all about it. It's very interesting. I went about, taught myself, I wasn't too unhappy, and then, honestly, I think it was February two years later, it went off like a bell in my head, and I thought "I can go to him now." And I cabled him. Of course at that time I also got into a difficulty with a patient, and I didn't know to whom to turn. I lived in Baltimore and I was the only analyst there. And then it went off: He said come, and why shouldn't I? So I cabled him, and went. So that's how that happened. And I think—certainly my analysis with him changed my personality quite definitely. I've had an analysis since then with Erich Fromm, which I think has given me much more solidity, but—well, each analysis has been very important at the level at which it happened. And I would say that xxxx xxx with Ferenczi it was almost 100% positive. Oh, I mean I can tell you what was wrong with it, but—

(Freud, 1952a, pp. 10–11)

This account adds a layer to the story of Sullivan, suggesting that Thompson should go into treatment with Ferenczi. As the story of the story goes, Sullivan thought Ferenczi was the only analyst he could learn from, and so he decided either he or Thompson should go to Ferenczi. The decision was made that it should be Thompson, and after her analysis, she should analyze Sullivan.

DR. E.: Yes, of course. What do you mean by what's wrong with it?

(Freud, 1952a, p. 11)

Finally, something strikes Eissler as interesting. This is the type of probing question he could have asked at many other times in the interview. Does he do it now because he is interested in finding fault with Ferenczi?

DR. T.: Well, I mean I can say what were the faults of my analyst in that; but certainly what he gave me was—I always thinking of Budapest as my, as reliving, as really growing up in a happy childhood—which was his fantasy about his method. But I really experienced it as that. Even to the fact that I didn't know what people were talking about around me—just like a child, it was, to live there in a country that was so foreign. And I think there were thirty-five Americans in all Budapest. Eight of those were my patients.

(Freud, 1952a, p. 11)

It is amazing that eight of her patients went with her to Budapest to continue their sessions. What does that mean about the nature of those relationships? If there were eight of them, Thompson was working quite a bit in Budapest, assuming she was seeing each of them three to five times per week while being in treatment with Ferenczi, four to five times a week.

Thompson cont'd
So that I was really in a foreign country. I think of it as a time in which I came to—I was a very detached person before that, very schizoid, and I came to have relationships with people for the first time. In a comfortable xxxxxxx social way. I still have difficulties with intimacy, although not too much. Silence:

(Freud, 1952a, p. 11)

This is someone—Thompson—who we believe means what she says. And so, when she writes about a change of this degree, we believe it. It's remarkable.

Of course, Freud figured greatly as the bad mother in my analysis.
DR. E.: Yes?
DR. T.: Yes. You see, my mother was the harsh one in my family. My father was very like Ferenczi, and so Freud was the bad mother, and I became very partisan in the whole fight.
DR. E.: Very what?
DR. T.: Very par—very much on Ferenczi's side, very much involved emotionally in his fight with Freud,—which I think I've gotten over.
DR. E.: But he must have spoken very often of Freud, probably also mentioned anecdotes, or some events, or—?

(Freud, 1952a, p. 11)

Thompson wants to tell Eissler that she played a part in the disturbance between Ferenczi and Freud, and beyond that, she offers an explanation that her participation with the two men was in part an extension of her own early family dynamics. But Eissler does not pursue this thread; instead, he focuses on what Ferenczi might have said about Freud.

DR. T.: Well, the ones I remember, those I've mentioned, the spitting, and about how often they walked together. That seemed to be a favorite way they had of discussing things, to walk in the mountains around Budapest or at, in Vienna, too. And apparently, oh, he felt also that Freud had stolen his ideas on homosexuality at the time—you see, what I'm talking about was the time when he was unhappy with Freud.

DR. E.: Yes.

(Freud, 1952a, p. 12)

Ferenczi thought Freud stole his ideas on homosexuality! The competition between Freud and Ferenczi was fierce, though Ferenczi is thought of as the person who conceded to Freud's authority. Ferenczi thought Freud stole his ideas about homosexuality. That may explain Freud's tempering of his position discussed earlier.

DR. T.: And I don't think that his happier times came to his mind so/ very much.

DR. E.: But when you met him here, in New York, he spoke about his relationship to Freud, or you heard it—?

DR. T.: I didn't know him. I only heard him speak at a lecture and I just talked to him once about my own analysis.

(Freud, 1952a, p. 12)

Eissler slides right past the accusation that Ferenczi felt Freud stole his ideas. He tries instead to direct Thompson to what Ferenczi might have said to her about Freud when they were in New York. But she explains how she did not know either man then. Her only contact with Ferenczi was about her own analysis.

DR. E.: Yes, but then you came in 1928, you first came—to analysis? (p. 12)

Again he reaches for something concrete.

DR. T.: Yes. (p. 12)

I wonder if Thompson becomes confused by Eissler's return to dates that have already been discussed.

DR. E.: And did he speak about Freud at that time?
DR. T.: No he didn't. (p. 12)

Eissler changes tactics and asks:

DR. E.: It would be interesting to compare his views, how they developed, xxx or how they changed from one year to another.
DR. T.: Yes. I wish I could, but I wasn't—I think xxx [1] wasn't enough in analysis at that time for him to talk about it, but it was at that time that he told me not to go and meet him, because he said he thought that Freud was very self-conscious with women about his appearance. Well, Freud did have some qualities of retiring, I guess.
DR. E.: I beg your pardon?
DR. T.: I said Freud did have some tendency to be withdrawn, as I recall.
DR. E.: Yes, he was—
DR. T.: But since I know so many people who did go from America and did meet him, I don't think he would have refused to see me.

Again, Eissler does not pursue what Thompson is telling him about Ferenczi keeping her from Freud.

DR. E.: Did he take new patients?
DR. T.: Who?
DR. E.: Freud.

(Freud, 1952a, pp. 12–13)

Here Thompson seems confused again. Are we talking about Ferenczi or Freud, she asks. It's as if she is saying, I'm telling you my experience and you seem to be focused on something else, something you want to hear. Thompson proceeds to tell Eissler some important facts about her relationship with Ferenczi and Freud's relationship with her friend Edith Jackson (see Chapter 5).

DR. T.: Well, Edith Jackson went, I think it must have been about 1929.

DR. E.: But she came as a patient, not as a visitor?

DR. T.: Yes, as a patient.

DR. E.: And you wanted to come as a visitor?

DR. T.: Yes, I wanted to—

DR. E.: And I don't know whether—

DR. T.: Maybe he didn't meet—

DR. E.: It was very difficult to meet Freud at that time. I never saw him.

(Freud, 1952a, p. 13)

Now we can understand Eissler a little better. He never met Freud; possibly, that is why he seems unsympathetic or uninterested in Thompson's wish to meet Freud.

DR. T.: Maybe it was a protective—

DR. E.: Yes. It is quite possible, yes.

DR. T.: And then I told you that he wrote on his birthday—Freud wrote on his birthday, which I think was either 1932 or 1931, that he hoped he wouldn't live another year, because he found life, he found his work was done and he found life nothing but a burden. Ferenczi read me that letter.

DR. E.: What did he say about that letter?

DR. T.: Well, he was very fond of Freud; that always stuck out throughout all of his unhappiness with him, and

DR. E.: And he worried that Freud wrote him that way, or—?

DR. T.: Well, he didn't worry; he felt sad about it, and it was in the same letter, I think, they were discussing some of Ferenczi's ideas. But he didn't really get angry with him, with Ferenczi, until towards the end. And I don't know—the paper that Ferenczi (1949) read at the Wiesbaden Congress[10]—Did you hear it?

DR. E.: No.

DR. T.: I heard it but it was in German, so I don't know. What I think the theme of this is, as Ferenczi told me, was his favorite theme; that there are no bad patients, there are only bad analysts, and tried to repeat the idea of the bad parent, making the neurotic child, and that the analyst can do the same sort of thing, can make the patient worse. Now, I don't know what else could have been in that paper but Freud was very disturbed about that paper, and that's the one he told him he must not publish, refused to let him publish, and I don't know whether it still exists or not.

DR. E.: Well the manuscript must exist. I must check. I always thought that the Wiesbaden paper was published. I will look once again.

DR. T.: I don't think it was published. No, I don't think it was. Ferenczi looked like death there. He was so white, it was startling when he sat on the platform with a row of ruddy-faced people who had been out in the sun. We should have realized how sick he was.

DR. E.: And—but then he read a paper in Vienna. That was published, I know—a xx years before he died. When was Wiesbaden?

DR. T.: Wiesbaden was nine months before he died.

DR. E.: Oh, then that must have been—I thought that Wiesbaden was before he read the paper—

DR. T.: No, Wiesbaden was the last paper he ever read; I'm sure because that—he became—that was when he became ill, while he was on that vacation, and he was brought home and he was quite ill all that winter.

(Freud, 1952a, pp. 13–14)

Thompson said in 1955, "The last paper that Ferenczi ever wrote, which was published for the first time in English in 1949 in the *International Journal*, was the Confusion of Tongues paper (see Thompson, 2017). The "Confusion of Tongues" paper (Ferenczi, 1949) is groundbreaking, but instead of exploring its significance, Thompson and Eissler resort to pinpointing dates. Thompson (1957) tells Fromm in a letter dated November 5, 1957 (housed in the Erich Fromm Archive, Tübingen) that "He [Ferenczi] was having a lot of trouble writing it [the paper] because he feared Freud would not approve."

DR. E.: He was treated for a while by Groddeck.[11] Do you know anything about that?

DR. T.: I know that he had a great admiration for Groddeck, and that I was in Baden-Baden with him one summer, 1929. He spent a month with Groddeck there. The month of September. And I imagine that they were—he was being treated by him, or something. He was, he had something of the same attitude towards Groddeck as he had towards Freud,—slightly contemptuous admiration for a powerful man. He showed him to me in the distance once, and he said, "Look at him, isn't he impressive?" And, yet there was, he would never quite admit that there was, he thought xxxxxxxxx—that is, Ferenczi thought the way Groddeck did. Although he greatly influenced his thinking, I'm sure.

DR. E.: Yes.

DR. T.: Groddeck made such tremendously extreme claims. I've always had great difficulty in following my analyst's enthusiasms. The trouble is—

DR. E.: Do you think that Groddeck exaggerated his therapeutic effects?

DR. T.: I don't see—it seems that they must have been exaggerated. I don't know.

DR. E.: Well, I grant you that I would never think that I would be able to achieve what Groddeck[12] got; on the other hand, I could imagine that someone who is a very powerful personality could actually reach that—such depths of—

DR. T.: Oh, yes, I suppose it is possible.

DR. E.: I mean one hears what may happen in hypnosis, or what happens in and those things xxx ᵃʳᵉ well documented.

(Freud, 1952a, pp. 14–15)

Here they are dancing around their beliefs.

DR. T.: Certainly Dr. Fromm-Reichmann was very much impressed with Groddeck.

DR. E.: Yes.

DR. T.: She was very much influenced by him. I think at the time that Ferenczi was so involved with him there was also the element of fighting Freud in there; that Groddeck was sort of an antagonist to Freud, at least in Ferenczi's thinking; and I think in most people's thinking. But apparently Ferenczi's always needed to have somebody as an authority beside him.

DR. E.: Well When Ferenczi was so sick, did he know what was wrong with him?

DR. T.: He told me it was pernicious anemia—I don't know—did he tell me? He knew he was sick, but I don't think he had any idea how sick he was.

DR. E.: And did he have an explanation for his sickness? Did he look at it psychologically, or how?

DR. T.: Yes, I think he felt—well, also he was rather bitter towards Mrs. La Verne, because apparently she had been analyzing him. He had been having dizzy spells for a long time, and they had been analyzing them as anxiety, and when they found what was really wrong, he was rather bitter towards, that he hadn't had any medical check-up on it. That's the trouble with analysts. Everything is psychic.

DR. E.: Mrs. La Verne made a real analysis?

DR. T.: I have no idea what went on between those two, but I think that he analyzed her one hour and she analyzed him the next—something like that. I think that—I think that he was completely afraid of her. For some reason it was—his wife felt that she bled him to death; his wife said this.

DR. E.: You knew Mrs. Ferenczi well?

DR. T.: Not too well. I knew her.

DR. E.: And what impression did you get of her?

DR. T.: I thought she was a very charming person; quite motherly and—I knew Elmo much better than the others.

DR. E.: His step-daughter.

DR. T.: Yes.

DR. E.: Did Mrs. Ferenczi tell you something about Freud?

DR. T.: No.

DR. E.: She never met him?

DR. T.: Yes, she knew Freud, certainly.

DR. E.: And Elmo met Freud?

DR. T.: I suppose so.

DR. E.: But she never mentioned him?

DR. T.: No. I never talked with them about Freud.

DR. E.: Would it be indiscreet if I asked you about what Ferenczi told you about his own childhood and youth? Or is that a personal question?

(Freud, 1952a, pp. 15–16)

An interesting question from Eissler, since he protected his own personal privacy.

DR. T.: Well, I don't know. I don't suppose the experiences of dead people xxx are too sacred after a number of years. He was a great reader apparently. His father had a bookstore in and he used to spend his time, he said, sitting on the top of the ladder in his father's book shop reading the books on the top shelves. He remembered the very early experience of—Is this right, or am I thinking of somebody else? Anyway, it seems to me that he said that he was put on a chamber and the chamber broke and cut him, and he remembered that as a very traumatic experience. He also apparently had a great problem with masturbation, and used to practice it to see if he could hit the ceiling with his semen in ejaculating. He had gonorrhea when he was 16, I think, which he got from a peasant girl. Now whether he ever had syphilis or not I don't know about it. There was all sorts of talk about it and I know that he was worried about paresis. He didn't marry and he was in love with Mrs. Ferenczi for many years before they were married. She didn't divorce her husband, and they had a child—she had a pregnancy which they had to get rid of. They never had any children after their marriage. She was quite a bit older than he, 7 or 8 years, I guess—or even more, because he told me he was nearer to the age of Elmo than he was to his wife's. You want to know all?

(Freud, 1952a, pp. 16–17)

At this point, one wonders why Thompson is revealing so much personal information about Ferenczi.

DR. E.: I beg your pardon?
DR. T.: Do you want to know about his love life?
DR. E.: Whatever—

(Freud, 1952a, p. 17)

Was Eissler disinterested? Perhaps he meant, "whatever you want to tell me." And, was either interrupted by Thompson or just trailed off. Elizabeth Severn did not reveal this kind of information about Ferenczi, in fact, she never said a disparaging thing about Ferenczi in her interview (Freud, 1952b).

DR. T.: He was in love with Elmo. He was—by the time he married Mrs. Ferenczi, he no longer loved her. He had fallen in love with her daughter, but she was so unhappy about it that he married her. And this seems to have been one of the tragedies of Elmo's, who seems to have had a very unhappy life. The other daughter, as you know, married Ferenczi's brother.

(Freud, 1952a, p. 17)

We learn from Berman (2004) that Elma Palos was Ferenczi's analysand, and then step-daughter and that these complex connections are important in understanding the Freud and Ferenczi's relationship. Freud and Ferenczi were both Elma's analyst and at Freud's urging, Ferenczi married Gizella

Palos, Elma's mother. Berman (2004) drawing from the correspondence of the participants in this drama provides an account of these complicated relationships, and Dupont (1995) explains how these private letters came into public hands. Thompson knows the story because Ferenczi told her.

DR. E.: No, I didn't know that.

DR. T.: So that he is the, he was the father-in-law of his brother and—it's rather complicated—anyway, a very mixed-up family situation. His brother died during the siege of Budapest.[13] His wife had her hands frozen so she could no longer use them.

DR. E.: That was in the Second World War?

DR. T.: Yes. During the siege. They lived in a cellar for nine weeks. Then she went to Switzerland, and she died there with Elmo. I think the other daughter is with Elmo now, too. Mrs. Kovac, I think, served as a kind of analyst to him from time to time. During his illness he talked quite a bit with Mrs. Kovac. I think he had quite a bit of hope that through analysis he would save himself from this pernicious anemia because he went on working very hard right after he had found out that he had it. Then I guess we have to give her credit for his getting rid of Mrs. La Verne.

DR. E.: Mrs. Kovac?

DR. T.: Yes. I know Freud sent of course all sorts of messages when he died.

DR. E.: I beg your pardon?

DR. T.: Freud sent all sorts of messages when he died. I didn't like his obituary of Ferenczi. He said he married too late in life. What did he mean by that? Remember, in the International?

DR. E.: Yes.

DR. T.: He said everything was because he married too late in life.

DR. E.: You said Freud sent all kinds of messages.

DR. T.: I don't know what they were but I know that the feeling was "Now it's too late," he seemed to be sorry.

DR. E.: But you had no opportunity of reading any of them?

DR. T.: No, I never read any of those. All of this I picked up unofficially, more or less, except that after Ferenczi was ill he talked—all of a sudden he talked much more in the last few months of his life. I suppose you would hardly say I had analysis.

(Freud, 1952a, pp. 17–18)

The fact that Thompson's analysis ended before Ferenczi's death is noteworthy. Ferenczi felt Thompson was more of a friend and colleague during the last months of his life. Thompson accepted on some level that her analysis had ended, and she and Ferenczi had entered a different phase of their relationship. She assumed they had terminated the analysis in the face of Ferenczi's impending death.

DR. E.: Did Fromm tell you about Freud?

DR. T.: I don't know whether Fromm knew Freud. Did Fromm know Freud?

DR. E.: No, but nevertheless—

DR. T.: No. I think he had definite theories about Freud's authoritarian character. I don't know whether he ever knew him personally or not.

DR. E.: And what did Fromm say of Ferenczi?

DR. T.: He thought that he was a very lovable person. Well, he agreed with me more or less about my feelings about his need for approval— Ferenczi's need for approval—and he thought, too, that maybe he was quite a conventional person basically. After all, he was a Hungarian. How could he help be impressed by/ pomp and ceremony?

DR. E.: That's correct. I think feudalism was quite deeply rooted in Hungary. A little bit more than in Austria. It was plenty in Austria, but in Hungary—

DR. T.: Yes. Because I wouldn't say that his basic character fits the picture at all. He was certainly not ostentatious himself in any way.

DR. E.: One would never think that—

DR. T.: But he was undoubtedly impressed with it.

DR. E.: There is a little movie in which Ferenczi is shown, and one gets the impression that he was a very simple person,

DR. T.: Yes. Is that the one with the little kid?

DR. E.: Yes.

DR. T.: Isn't that lovely? It's so like him, yes.

DR. E.: It's extremely appealing. One gets immediately this when one sees him.

DR. T.: Oh, yes. You love this man almost at once.

DR. E.: Sometimes in talking about all those things, new memories come back, little trivial details, which may be quite important.

DR. T.: I remember his dog got hold of a bird one time, and he was very upset by that, and got the bird away from the dog. And xxxxx then was very upset because the bird died.

DR. E.: Did he say anything about Freud's relationship to dogs?

DR. T.: No. Of course I've heard a lot about that from others, but I

DR. E.: Yes, you did?

DR. T.: Well, I mean I've seen the pictures, and I know—Edith Jackson told me—she has one of Freud's dogs—and the idea that dogs were always present at the analysis of people, I've heard. I know—I've ana- lyzed one of the children, of the people who were analyzed as a child by Anna Freud, and one of her grievances was that there was always the dog there, as if she never had Anna all to herself.[14]

DR. E.: The dog was also in Anna's room?

DR. T.: Yes. I don't know whether it was the same dog. There were several dogs there.

DR. E.: I think there were two.

DR. T.: Yes. Well one was always lying in Anna's room, by the couch apparently.

DR. E.: Did you hear from that child anything more?

DR. T.: I don't think she had much to do with him. Judith de Forest[15]— she's an analyst now—she was the child that I analyzed. She lived with Dorothy Burlingham, she boarded with her during, I think, one year that she was away from her mother, in her adolescence. Her memory of this year was great deprivation, a feeling of great lack of warmth. Now, whether this was her neurosis—which it was also—or whether there was a rather cold atmosphere in Dorothy Burlingham's house, I don't know. She is not a cold person now. Judith de Forest is certainly not a cold person now. She's a pretty happy person, I think.

DR. E.: Did Ferenczi mention anything about Freud's family?

DR. T.: He was very fond of Anna, and one day he said, "Such a wonderful woman wasted." He seemed to feel that—well, I guess we all feel it— that her attachment to her father was such that she could never marry, she could never find anybody as good as her father. It just was a great waste. He thought she was a very feminine person, she should have found love in marriage. I know he was very fond of her.

(Freud, 1952a, pp. 18–20)

Does Thompson look back on her own life and see her choice not to marry as a shortcoming, or are these comments solely about Anna Freud?

DR. E.: And about Mrs. Freud—did he mention her?

DR. T.: I don't remember his mentioning her, anything about her.

DR. E.: And the other children?

DR. T.: No, I've never heard anything about them.

DR. E.: Did he ever tell you about rumors, gossip, regarding Freud? Second-hand information?

DR. T.: No, I don't remember any.

DR. E.: Or certain ideas he had, things he thought about Freud, and so on?

DR. T.: Only those that I've told you: about his feeling that Freud really despised patients, otherwise not. I'm afraid Freud figured in most of our conversation much more as my bad mother xx than as a person.

(Freud, 1952a, p. 20)

Thompson compares her disapproving mother to the dynamics between Ferenczi and Freud.

DR. E.: Yes. But that's why it makes it so important because it is an aspect which one hears rarely. Therefore, it would be so important to hear as much as possible from you.

DR. T.: Well, I had a great difficulty with a rigid mother, who was very religious and very—she was really a very frightened person but she covered it up with this controlling rigidity: "You must do this and you mustn't do that." And there was something in Freud's thinking that fit into this, which I immediately xxxxx fastened on to. Especially so much of Ferenczi's attitude was like my father's in that, "Oh, that you must understand him" in the early part of my analysis to try to see him in this setting than to xxx to be hostile to him, so that we worked out the drama very well, except that it wasn't my family. Then Mrs. La Verne became a much better bad mother than Freud.

(Freud, 1952a, p. 20)

Thompson's mother was hostile and abusive to her, while she found Ferenczi to be more like her father, who was kind and perhaps supportive. She intensely disliked Elizabeth Severn.

DR. E.: He spoke about Mrs. La Verne directly or you heard about her?

DR. T.: Well I met her. I saw her quite often.

DR. E.: But I mean did he tell you something about her?

DR. T.: Yes, he did tell me quite a bit about her. It's uncanny. I had an uncanny experience in that I've had three analysts and they've all been involved with women who had a great deal of hypochondriasis. I had an analyst before Ferenczi, a totally unknown American—a man named Joe Thompson. He's dead now. He married a patient who also had the same kind of weird childhood memories. Mrs. La Verne and this other woman also reconstructed the most sadistic sexual accomplishments having been perpetrated on them as children. Now they were almost identical, those stories, so that this must be something that x goes on in that type of person.

DR. E.: Yes.

DR. T.: All kinds of tortures, of having been tied in their beds and beaten and so forth, which seems to have been—I put Eric Fromm in here now because of his wife's having been ill so long. But maybe she was more ill than we realized.

(Freud, 1952a, pp. 20–21)

Thompson is referring to three women (Fromm's second wife, Henny Gurland Fromm, Joseph Chessman Thompson's wife, Anna Thompson, and Elizabeth Severn) who she knew personally including their hypochondriacal symptoms and their related sexual trauma with what sounds like, little empathy. Her use of language (i.e., "sexual accomplishments" as opposed to sexual abuse) is unusual. This may be a remnant of language from another era. Thompson uses the word "accomplishments" to signify deeds or actions. But as Brennan (2015) has opined, "Thompson had a lot of experience working with very sick patients, including many psychotics, so her reaction to the depth of Severn's suffering is striking, and the tone sounds like one of skepticism" (p. 88). Why doesn't she concern herself with their suffering? Should we conclude that this is a dissociative response and evidence of her having been sexually abused as is described in Ferenczi's diary (Dupont, 1988, p. 3). Sometimes the easiest assumptions can mislead (see Chapter 4).

Ferenczi was collaborating with Thompson to theorize sexual trauma and childhood trauma generally. The collaborative working through of Severn's sexual trauma by Severn, Ferenczi, and Thompson led to the development of new techniques in psychoanalysis and to a theory of trauma (Rachman, 2018, Rachman & Klett, 2018.). But Thompson in her own work stayed away from the topic. Her statement, "I am a pupil of

Ferenczi for over ten years I have made use of some of his techniques in my psycho-analytic work. In the course of time, I have discarded several of his ideas and confirmed the validity of others. . . I believe that Ferenczi pointed out things in need of emphasis in the analytic world. He was the only person in Europe at the time who saw some of them, and had the courage to state them." Thompson (1943, p. 64) suggests that she was fully aware of all his ideas but chose to utilize only some.

DR. E.: Did Ferenczi mention other disagreements with Freud besides theory?

DR. T.: No, I think his basic disagreement was this about being too harsh with patients.

DR. E.: Technical questions? But did he tell you something about what Freud said about the Thalasa, for example?

DR. T.: Well, he said that Freud liked that very much and thought that was a great book. I know Freud rather played down the Ice Age.[16] Ferenczi himself said, "that was a great fantasy of mine."

DR. E.: But Freud accepted it?

DR. T.: Yes. Freud accepted that. I think that was one of the last things that he wrote that Freud accepted. Well that was right at the transition point. He published that just as he started on his relaxation career.

DR. E.: Yes. But you don't remember particular opinions Freud had about specific papers of Ferenczi?

DR. T.: No. I don't think I ever heard any. I know that Ferenczi liked Death[17]—his stages in the ^ development of the sense of reality. That, he felt, was his stroke of genius. I think it's a pretty fine paper myself.

DR. E.: It's an excellent paper. Do you remember that Freud said anything about that paper?

DR. T.: No, I don't recall whether he did or not.

DR. E.: Did Ferenczi work with hypnosis?

DR. T.: He must have earlier. His paper on Transference certainly seems to imply a man who knew a lot about hypnosis and I think he did. In fact I think it says so in the International Journal, that he did quite a bit of hypnosis. I imagine he did the mother type, as he describes it, who could never be stern.

DR. E.: Did he tell you something about his early meetings with Freud, the impressions he got?

DR. T.: No, he didn't talk to me about that. That I got also out of the International Journal, what little I know about it.

DR. E.: And the years when he was in the army, do you know something about that?

DR. T.: No.

DR. E.: There's one reference in Freud that he tried to lecture to officers but—about the Oedipus Complex—but he quickly discontinued his lecture. The happy days were over.

DR. T.: Ferenczi had a brief period during the Communist Revolution of being a professor, I think, it was at the University.

DR. E.: Yes.

DR. T.: And he was very frightened of Hitler, you see he died soon after he came to power. And I know all that last year he was talking about we must go and find an island somewhere. We would all go to an island somewhere. I being an American couldn't take all this too seriously. It never occurred to me that there was danger in the world at that time. But he was very anxious, apparently felt that Europe was doomed, and he seems to have been right. I know there was a railroad wreck, a train wreck in Hungary in about 1932, I guess, or 1931 which was produced by a maniac who derailed—the man was later picked up in Vienna. He apparently was a pervert who produced wrecks and stood by and masturbated while he saw the people die. Well, at first it was in the midst of all this unrest, and the first thought about this wreck was that it was a Hitler thing, the Nazis. Then even I got a little alarmed, but then they soon found this man.

DR. E.: And did Ferenczi say something about that?

DR. T.: Well, I don't think he thought it was the Nazis. I'm just saying that somehow his anxiety finally lighted something in me so that when the train wreck came I got really anxious.

DR. E.: Did he have a discussion with Freud about such political things? The future of Europe

DR. T.: I don't know.

DR. E.: Do you remember anything he said about the future of psychoanalysis, how it would develop, what standing it would have as a therapy?

DR. T.: Well, I don't think that he, Ferenczi, was as interested as to what standing it would have in society as he was always interested in his working out a technique that would work. That certainly was what his whole relaxation study he thought was going to make it really good, make people cured. That all they needed was to get the love they'd never had, and then they'd get well. I don't know why Ferenczi doesn't seem to have been influenced by the growing trend of character analysis more than he was.

DR. E.: Well I think character analysis was—well, I mean xxxxxxx ^ if you want to translate into analytic terms—really an attack against the patient. Reich x really called it pain,⁷ and I could imagine that it was incompatible with his strong feeling for mankind.

DR. T.: Yes, I guess that's probably it.

DR. E.: A really relentless attack against the patient. Did you remember that he said anything about it? about how he—

DR. T.: No, he didn't. That's why I said I didn't know anything about xxx ^Reich's work until I came back to the United States, and then his book had just been published in German. The first winter I was here in New York, after I came back, and I remember we had some—a little group of us met and discussed it. And to me this was a—not that I would ever have been able to use the aggression that he did—but to me it was a great new, a whole new insight about the way to deal with personality; which I would say was the one thing Ferenczi never did meet. He never actually had any conception of my character structure. Certainly he dealt plenty with my traumatic experiences and with my relationships to people, but the ways in which my hostility was expressed I don't think he ever saw. The ways in which I manipulated people, I am sure he never saw.

(Freud, 1952a, pp. 21–24)

Thompson confirms that Ferenczi dealt with her traumatic experiences. The trauma she mentions in the *Clinical Diary* is the physical abuse she suffered at the hands of her mother.

DR. E.: Yes. That's strange because he resented that Freud had neglected that in his analysis, and xxxx ^some people, I mean, are particularly observant of that which was neglected in their own analysis because they want to match up. But you think he had no feeling for that particular aspect?

DR. T.: Well I don't think he saw his own need of love as a neurosis. I think that's where he missed out. I think that's where his whole relaxation therapy missed out, in that he really thought that you could give an adult the love he never had, which you can't, because it's shut off.

(Freud, 1952a, p. 24)

This is an important point of disagreement between Thompson and Ferenczi.

DR. E.: Yes.

DR. T.: And he didn't see this, that actually the character has developed a rigidity against love by the time they have grown up, and that no matter how much you feed them, it's just like diabetes; the sugar isn't digested.

DR. E.: Is it something that you then became aware of after you—

DR. T.: Yes. I got that in my analysis with Fromm. But I also became aware of it before my analysis, I mean from reading Reich.[18] I got a lot of ideas from that.

(Freud, 1952a, p. 24)

The termination of Thompson's analysis with Ferenczi coincided with his fatal illness. Ferenczi was able to say his farewells and acknowledge that she was an important person to him. He requested that she, "his best pupil," continue his work. Her goodbye was difficult. She could not utter the words.

We leave this interview having met Clara Thompson. A woman who courageously sailed to a foreign country to enter psychoanalysis with Freud's Hungarian disciple, Sándor Ferenczi. A pioneering psychoanalyst who emerged from her analysis with Ferenczi having shaken up the status quo of Freudian psychoanalysis, ultimately becoming the anointed heir of Ferenczi's innovative treatment techniques. She went on to develop an American psychoanalysis as the esteemed Director of the William Alanson White Institute in New York, the home of the Interpersonal Psychoanalytic tradition.

Moments That Stand Out

Thompson, like many psychoanalysts at the time, had a desire to meet Freud, and Ferenczi had a role in thwarting that effort. There was an intimacy between Thompson and Ferenczi, reflected in how open he was with her about his personal life and his willingness to collaborate with her around the treatment of another analysand, Elizabeth Severn. There was the hint of a backstory involving Thompson's communication with

Edith Jackson, Freud's analysand, and her wish for Ferenczi to stand up to Freud about his new techniques that was embedded in the story of her kissing her analyst, Ferenczi. And then there is Thompson's criticism of Elizabeth Severn for her perceived misuse of Ferenczi's kindness. There is also a troubling point in the interview where Thompson speaks of Ferenczi's sexually abused patients in what sounds like at minimum an intellectualized and detached—or worse, dissociated—manner. It is also associated with her befuddlement over whether the "Confusion of Tongues" (Ferenczi, 1949) paper was published. These points reemerge in the following chapters.

Throughout the interview, we hear Thompson's non-aggressive persistence as she steers the interview in the direction that she, not Eissler, chooses. She tells her story, despite Eissler wanting to hear a story about Freud. The rhythm of the interview is inconsistent as topics appear and reappear as Thompson persists in making her voice heard. We learn of her willingness to believe Ferenczi was ashamed of her despite how she also learned that he felt she was his best pupil. This apparent diffidence in Thompson's personality can be partly understood as a characteristic of her New England heritage.

Throughout her life, she showed humility rather than conceit—more in line with the theological concept of divine grace, an individual virtue rather than weakness. She can be formidable without intimidating others. All these contradictions are part and parcel of the Thompson we meet in this interview and the Thompson that comes to life in the following biographical narrative, as she weathers the storms of life's transitions, ensuing professional psychoanalytic battles, personal losses, and stunning achievements.

Notes

1 Ferenczi's (1933) Confusion of tongues between adults and children: The language of tenderness and passion. Presented first at the Wiesbaden Congress 1932 offered a new theory of trauma.

2 This interview appears here without any editorial emendations, typographical corrections, deletions, altered punctuation, or ellipses in compliance with the requirements as stated by Dr. Emanuel E. Garcia, the literary executor of the K.R. Eissler Estate. Thank you to Louis Rose, Executive Director, Sigmund Freud Archives, Professor of Modern European History, Department of History, Otterbein University, Westerville, OH for assisting in the use of the interview.

3 Elizabeth Severn is sometimes referred to as Mrs. La Verne in the interview.
4 Pernicious anemia is a rare blood disorder characterized by the inability of the body to properly utilize vitamin B12, which is essential for the development of red blood cells.
5 Rachman (1997) points out that the Nobel prize had been awarded for a synthesis of a new drug to treat anemia that was not available to Ferenczi.
6 An interview with Dr. Zeborah Schachtel dated October, 2016.
7 This was relevant if there was a case of neurosyphilis.
8 The psychoanalyst Helene Deutsch born in Poland immigrated to the United States in 1935. Publishing in 1925, she specialized in the psychology of women staying close to Freud's main theories.
9 The psychoanalyst Esther Menaker travelled to Vienna in 1930 to train as a psychoanalyst at the Vienna Psychoanalytic Institute. Her first analyst was Anna Freud. She embraced ego psychology focusing on preoedipal dynamics and their influence in shaping subjectivity within the mother–infant dyad. She published more than 45 articles and 6 books.
10 Ferenczi presented his paper *Confusion of Tongues* on the first day of the Wiesbaden Congress, Friday, September 2, 1932. Freud sent a telegram to Ettingon condemning the paper; Freud also tried to suppress the paper's publication.
11 Georg Groddeck is a Swiss psychoanalytically oriented physician known as the pioneer of psychosomatic medicine. He was a friend of Sigmund Freud's and Sándor Ferenczi and director of the spa/sanatorium at Baden-Baden.
12 This note inserted into the interview without a page number reads: Note: Dr. Thompson, I believe, was expressing the idea that Ferenczi would never quite admit that he himself thought the way Grodeck Thought.] Maxine L. Rippner (Transcriber of Interview)
13 The Siege of Budapest was a 50-day long encirclement by Soviet forces of Budapest. Nearly 40,000 civilians died through starvation or military action beginning December 24, 1944 and lasting till the city surrendered February 13, 1945.
14 Thompson is referring to Judith Brasher de Forest, the daughter of Alfred and Izette de Forest, who was analyzed by Thompson following her analysis with Anna Freud.
15 Judith de Forest's father Alfred was a cousin of Dorothy Tiffany Burlingham. This connection brought the de Forest and Burlingham households together with the Freuds. Judy de Forest spent a year and a half with the Burlinghams in Vienna, where she was in analysis with Anna Freud (Brennan, 2009).
16 In *Thalassa* Ferenczi presented his theory that civilization was a reaction to the catastrophe of the ice age (Ferenczi, 1938).
17 His theory concerning a connection between death throes and sexual excitement, is discussed in Ferenczi (1938).
18 Wilhelm Reich was an Austrian psychoanalyst who combined psychoanalysis with Marxism. The book Thompson was referring to is *Character Analysis*

(1933). He also published *The Mass Psychology of Fascism* (1933) and *Sexual Revolution* (1936).

References

Abelove, H. (1993). Freud, male homosexuality, and the Americans. In H. Abelove, M. A. Barale, & D. Halperin (Eds.), *The lesbian and gay studies reader* (pp. 381–393). Routledge.

Bergler, E. (1939). On the psychoanalysis of the ability to wait and of impatience. *Psychoanalytic Review, 26*(1), 11–32.

Bergler, E. (1940). Four types of neurotic indecisiveness. *Psychoanalytic Quarterly, 9*(4), 481–492.

Bergler, E. (1956). *Homosexuality: Disease or way of life.* Hill & Wang.

Berman, E. (2004). Sándor, Gizella, Elma: A biographical journey. *International Journal of Psychoanalysis, 85*(2), 489–520.

Bonomi, C. (1999). Flight into sanity: Jones's allegation of Ferenczi's mental deterioration reconsidered. *International Journal of Psychoanalysis, 80*(3), 507–542.

Brennan, B. W. (2015). Out of the archive/Unto the couch: Clara Thompson's analysis with Ferenczi. In A. Harris & S. Kuchuck (Eds.), *The legacy of Sándor Ferenczi: From ghost to ancestor* (pp. 77–95). Routledge.

Drescher, J. (1996). Psychoanalytic subjectivity and male homosexuality. In R. P. Cabaj & T. S. Stein (Eds.), *Textbook of homosexuality and mental health* (pp. 173–189). American Psychiatric Press.

Drescher, J. (1997). From preoedipal to postmodern: Changing psychoanalytic attitudes toward homosexuality. *Gender and Psychoanalysis, 2*(2), 203–216.

Drescher, J. (2008). A history of homosexuality and organized psychoanalysis. *Journal of the American Academy of Psychoanalysis and Dynamic Psychiatry, 36*(3), 443–460.

Dupont, J. (Ed.). (1988). *The clinical diary of Sándor Ferenczi* (M. Balint & N. Z. Jackson, Trans.). Harvard University Press.

Dupont, J. (1995). The story of transgression. *Journal of American Psychoanalytic Association, 43*, 823–834.

Eisold, K. (2018). *The organizational life of psychoanalysis: Conflicts, dilemmas, and the future of the profession.* Routledge.

Falzeder, E., Brabant, E., & Giampieri-Deutsch, P. (Eds.). (2000). *The correspondence of Sigmund Freud and Sándor Ferenczi (Volume 3, 1920–1933)* (P. T. Hoffer, Trans.). Harvard University Press.

Ferenczi, S. (1932). "The passions of adults and their influence on the sexual and character development of children." Paper presentation in German.

Ferenczi, S. (1934) Gedanken über das Trauma: Aus dem Nachlaß von. Internationale Zeitschrift für Psychoanalyse 20:5–12. Later as, Ferenczi, S. (1949) Confusion of tongues between adults and children: the language of tenderness and passion. International *Journal of Psychoanalysis*, 30, 225–230. And also as Ferenczi, S. (1988) Confusion of Tongues between Adults and the Child, Contemporary Psychoanalysis, 24:2, 196–206, DOI: 10.1080/00107530.1988.10746234.

Ferenczi, S. (1926). The problem of acceptance of unpleasant ideas: Advances in knowledge of the sense of reality. *International Journal of Psychoanalysis*, 7:312–323

Ferenczi, S. (1934) Thalassa: A Theory of Genitality, The Psychoanalytic Quarterly, 3:1, 1–29, DOI: 10.1080/21674086.1934.11925198

Ferenczi, S. (1949). Confusion of tongues between adults and the child (The language of tenderness and of passion). *International Journal of Psychoanalysis*, *30*, 225–230.

Freud, S. (1935). Anonymous (Letter to an American mother). In E. Freud (Ed.), *The letters of Sigmund Freud* (pp. 423–424). Basic Books.

Freud, S. (1952a). *Interview with Clara Thompson (K. R. Eissler, Interviewer)*. Manuscript/Mixed Material. Sigmund Freud Papers: Interviews and Recollections, Set A, 1914–1998 (Box 122). Manuscripts Division, Library of Congress, Washington, DC. www.loc.gov/item/mss3999001575/

Freud, S. (1952b). *Interview with Dr. Elizabeth Severn, December 20, 1952. (K. R. Eissler, Interviewer)*. Manuscript/Mixed Material. Sigmund Freud Papers: Interviews and Recollections, Set A, 1914–1998 (Box 122). Manuscripts Division, Library of Congress, Washington, DC. www.loc.gov/item/mss3999001567/

Fromm, E. (1964). Foreword. In M. R. Green (Ed.), *Interpersonal psychoanalysis: The selected papers of Clara M. Thompson.* (pp. v,vi) Basic Books.

Green, M. R. (Ed.). (1964). *Interpersonal psychoanalysis: The selected papers of Clara M. Thompson.* Basic Books.

Jones, E. (1953). *The life and work of Sigmund Freud, Volume 3: The last phase 1919–1939.* Basic Books.

Malcolm, J. (2000, January 2). The lives they lived: Kurt Eissler, b. 1908; Keeper of Freud's secrets. *The New York Times Magazine.* www.nytimes.com/2000/01/02/magazine/the-lives-they-lived-kurt-eissler-b-1908-keeper-of-freud-s-secrets.html

Masson, J. M. (1985). *The assault on truth: Freud's suppression of the seduction theory.* Penguin Books.

Menaker, E. (1989). *Appointment in Vienna: An American psychoanalyst recalls her student days in pre-war Austria.* St. Martin's Press.

Rachman, A. W. (1997). *Sándor Ferenczi: The psychotherapist of tenderness and passion.* Jason Aronson.

Rachman, A. W. (2018). *Elizabeth Severn: The "evil genius" of psychoanalysis.* Routledge.

Rachman, A. W., & Klett, S. A. (2018). Analysis of the Incest Trauma: Retrieval, recovery, renewal. Routledge.

Reich, W. (1945) *Character Analysis*, Farrar, Straus and Giroux, New York.

Sankovitch, N. (2017). *The Lowells of Massachusetts*. St. Martin's Press.

Stern, D. B. (2019). *The infinity of the unsaid: Unformulated experience, language, and the nonverbal*. Routledge.

Thompson, C. (1943). The therapeutic technique of Sándor Ferenczi: A comment. *International Journal of Psychoanalysis*, *24*, 64–66.

Thompson, C. (1944). Ferenczi's contribution to psychoanalysis. *Psychiatry*, *7*(3), 245–252.

Thompson, C. (1947). Changing concepts of homosexuality in psychoanalysis. *Psychiatry*, *10*, 183–189.

Thompson, C. (1957, November 5). Letter to Erich Fromm. Housed in the Erich Fromm Archive, Tübingen.

Thompson, C. (1958). A study of the emotional climate of psychoanalytic institutes. *Psychiatry*, *21*(1), 45–51. (Original paper presented at the December 1957 meeting of the William Alanson White Psychoanalytic Society)

Thompson, C. (2017) The history of the William Alanson White Institute. Contemporary Psychoanalysis, 53:1, 7–28.

Chapter 2

Early Life and Education
From Conformist to Rebel

A Rebel

Clara Mabel Thompson was born in 1893 in Providence, Rhode Island, a city resting at the outlet of the Providence River and the Narragansett Bay. It is one of the oldest cities in the country and founded by Rodger Williams, a reformed Baptist theologian who was forced to leave the Massachusetts Bay Colony because of his radical ideas. It is in the politics and culture of Providence that Thompson's worldviews were initially formed. Her family and the schools she attended were steeped in religious ideas of salvation, liberal philosophies, and limited—beliefs in civil rights and equality—that merged with the then-dominant American ethics of pragmatism and self-realization. This complex cultural legacy was pivotal in the life choices of this pioneering psychoanalyst. As she wrote:

> [O]ne learns to fit into the life to which he is born without ever knowing that he is missing something. It is only by comparison with other situations, such as another culture, another group, or another family, that one may get the feeling of frustration in some areas. The individual is truly a product of his culture as brought to him, first through his parents and later through his other life opportunities. Only rarely does there occur a maverick, one whose life experiences somehow made him a rebel rather than a conformist. But even then, the degree of his deviation is not permitted to be unlimited. Beyond a certain point, society forbids his deviation, and few can survive that degree of disapproval.
>
> (Thompson, 1958, p. 13)

DOI: 10.4324/9781003261797-3

Clara Thompson was a product of her culture, a culture that was both religiously restrictive and encouraging through self-realization, an effort encouraged initially as a way to become close to God.

317 Jastram Street

Clara Lois Medbury[1] (1868–1952) and Thomas Frank Thompson (1864–1930) were 20 and 24 when they married in Providence, Rhode Island, in 1888. As a wedding present, their parents pooled their resources to build the young couple a large white clapboard house at 317 Jastram Street, with double porches that hung over the entrance. When their first child, Clara Mabel Thompson, was born five years later, on October 3, 1893, her mother possibly thought that her namesake daughter would be just like her. The family called the young Clara "Mabel," an innocent familial tactic to avoid confusion. A second child, Frank Jr., followed seven years later, in 1900. By that time, both sets of grandparents, along with an assortment of relatives, had moved into the home (Green, 1964). The house may have seemed like a good financial arrangement, but it was also the case that for both sets of parents, their religion viewed the family as "an agent of godly living" and advocated for all family members to reside in one household.

While we know from Sprague (2011) that Thompson's maternal grandfather sold vegetables and was a lamplighter for the city, Green (1964) explains that Clara—Mabel—was drawn to the paternal side of the family. He points out that as a young child Thompson came into conflict with her mother and maternal grandmother, turning her away from the Medbury side of the family. Her interest was in the Swedish-born paternal side of the family which she saw as more adventurous and creative and less conforming. For a time, her paternal grandfather worked on a whaling ship. Her paternal grandmother loved to paint pictures of the sea. (Green, 1964). According to Sprague (2011), her paternal grandmother was the source of stories about her grandfather whose death occurred sometime before she was born. The tales her grandmother told her about her grandfather's exploits might well have inspired her enduring love of the ocean and sense of adventure and ignited her yearning for freedom.

There are two different and deep sources of biographical information on Clara Mabel Thompson. The first is by Maurice Green (1964) who provided vital information that at this point would otherwise be impossible to find.

We are all indebted to him for his biographical essay. I have also drawn on the discussion of Clara Thompson's early life in Elizabeth Capelle's 1993 dissertation, *"Analyzing the 'Modern Woman': Psychoanalytic Debates About Feminism, 1920–1950."* Her discussion of the role of the Free Will Baptists in Thompson's life as well as her later position on feminism has been essential. Capelle's work provides a more nuanced picture of Clara Thompson and what it meant for a young woman of her era to aspire to become a medical missionary. In another instance, Capelle elaborates on what it might have meant for Thompson to identify with the protagonist, Maggie, in *The Mill on the Floss*. Like Thompson, the fictional character suffered a harsh and rejecting mother.

From Green (1964) we learn that as a young child she tried to imitate her paternal grandmother and that too could have caused tension between the young Mabel and her mother. Clara Thompson's mother came from a long lineage of New England stock. The Rhode Island Historical Society dates the Medbury family as far back as 1654. Religion formed the core of her mother's identity and community. The elder Clara was an Evangelical Baptist Sunday school teacher, who is consistently described as "religious" (Capelle, 1993; Green, 1964). She was also harsh, critical, demanding, and abusive. She openly favored Clara's younger brother, Frank Jr., reportedly because her husband favored their daughter. In a painful tale told in Sándor Ferenczi's *Clinical Diary* (Dupont, 1988), Thompson reveals that her mother once pulled young Clara's arm so roughly that she broke it. Thompson's retelling of that trauma occurred during a psychoanalytic session with Ferenczi. She later attributed her mother's abusive behavior to the fact that her mother was an extremely anxious person who tried to control everyone around her. Thompson confided to her close friend, the psychoanalyst Zeborah Schachtel, that when she looked into her mother's eyes, she experienced a "terrible feeling of coldness" (Zeborah Schachtel, personal communication, 2018). That description aligns with Green's (1964) characterization of Thompson's mother as "rigid" and gives depth to our understanding of the complexities of their relationship. Thompson felt compelled to silence her true feelings to avoid conflict with her mother.

Clara Thompson adored her father. Her father Frank began his career as a tailor and then took a job as a traveling salesman for a drug company. He was ambitious and rose in the ranks to become the president of the successful Blanding Pharmaceutical Company, which still exists to this day, advertising itself to be the oldest pharmaceutical company in the country. Described by a friend of Thompson as a "handsome" man, Frank was seen as someone who "held his head proudly" and who had a "quick and penetrating" look, with a mustache "flying from his face" (Green, 1964, p. 351). Although he attended weekly church services with the family, the elder Frank was more invested in his career than in religion. Unlike his wife, the extent of his involvement in devout practices most likely stopped at church services.

Despite the families' commonalities, the Thompson/Medbury household was a place of considerable tension. The major source of conflict was the differences in religious dedication. Although both sides of the family were Free Will Baptists, the Thompsons were less conforming to religious ideology and practice, compared with the maternal Medbury side, who were much more devout. While the Thompsons likely participated in festive meals and regular Sunday services, the Medburys were more strictly adherent to scripture as well as more deeply involved with the religion's organizational and community life, including bake sales, suppers, sewing circles, and Sunday school. The Medburys adhered more strictly to Baptist prohibitions that forbade dancing, drinking, and sex before marriage. Their attitudes toward gender behavior followed conventional biblical scripture. By contrast, the Thompsons kept a distance from such religious fervor. These differences divided the household, causing interpersonal friction. Despite this, when they attended the Jefferson Street Baptist church, they no doubt presented the picture of a cohesive family.

Even during vacations, Clara Thompson's family was tethered to their religious community. The family spent time during the summer in Orchard Beach, Maine, near the site of the Free Will Baptist revival camp in Ocean Park. This historic camp, located down the beach from central Old Orchard, is just outside of Portland. Built in the late 1800s by Oren B. Cheney, the president of Bates College, its mission was to establish a summer resort where religious, educational, and other meetings could be held.

Green (1964) reports that Mabel was a dutiful child and an outstanding honors student, as well as a "typical American tomboy" (p. 349) who was popular with other children. She liked outdoor sports and competitive athletic games. She liked to play with the boys as they all explored the wooded areas around Providence (Green, 1964).

But, to Thompson's mother, her daughter's high-spirited nature and tomboy behavior were a growing affront to her sense of what was acceptable behavior for a young Free Will Baptist girl. While Thompson's felt experience of her family's religious practices was mostly limited to attending church and Sunday school during her primary school years, things changed dramatically as she approached adolescence. That's when her mother began pressing Thompson with demands to conform to what was expected of her. From that point on, being a tomboy was no longer acceptable. Her tomboy behavior was met with a push to adhere to the conventions of femininity: cooperativeness, modesty, humility, and tenderness; being kind, helpful, and understanding were values that were expected. Gone was Thompson's guiltless pleasure in playing competitive sports with the neighborhood boys and girls. Instead, prohibitions were instated against aggression, the pleasures of dancing, and a mandate to be chaste. In later years she often "delighted in telling how she had splashed indecorously around in the baptismal pool" when she was baptized by total immersion at age twelve— "she had to be hauled out forcibly when the solemn ritual was over" (Green, 1964, p. 349). The story attests to both her spirited and rebellious nature that began in childhood and her enduring love of the water. Sprague (2011) notes that her "happy immersion stood for her overall approach to life. She did not take to things partially or tepidly. She immersed" (p. 38).

From 1908 to 1912, Clara Thompson attended Classical High School in Providence, a prestigious preparatory public school. She was a serious student who ranked at the head of her class in all her academic subjects and participated in extracurricular activities including basketball and the Christian Endeavor group, a youth church group that stressed devotion and an evangelical spirit. Fellowship activities included things like hiking and birdwatching, but the goal of the group is best understood by the pledge members took, which begins:

> Trusting in the Lord Jesus Christ for strength, I promise Him that I will strive to do whatever He would like to have me do; that I will make it the rule of my life to pray and to read the Bible every day, and to support the work and worship of my own church in every way possible; and that just so far as I know how, throughout my whole life, I will endeavor to lead a Christian life.
>
> (World's Christian Endeavor Union)

At Classical High School, she led the girls' debate team—that proved early training for the many vigorous arguments and discussions she would participate in later in her professional life. Because of her stellar academic record, she was chosen as one of her class's commencement speakers.

Classical High School was a serious learning environment whose motto was taken from a Tennyson poem: "To Strive, to Seek, to Find, and Not to Yield." Thompson took these words to heart. She was a committed and curious student across a wide range of subjects. In her 1912 high school yearbook, she is described by her classmates as:

> one of those naturally bright people one reads about in books. Trans-lation of Virgil or Homer or, indeed, studying in general is no trouble for her. As president of the G.D.S. [Girl's Debating Society] she is a very important and influential member, while basketball claims her every Friday. Her hopes for the future are uncommon and ambi-tious. When we hear of her work as a doctor among the women of India, we shall all look at each other proudly and say, "She was our classmate." . . . Here's metal most attractive, wearing all that weight of learning lightly.
>
> (Green, 1964, p. 350)

The reference to Thompson as someone who would "work as a doctor administering to the women of India" reflected her emerging plan to become a medical missionary, a plan she announced during one of the meetings of her Christian Endeavor group (Capelle, 1993). Missionary work may have had the appeal of combining a life of service with a life of adventure. For a young woman like Clara Thompson becoming a medical missionary may have been viewed as an alternative to marriage. Becoming a medical missionary would have pleased her mother while also allowing her to follow her desire to become a physician. This medical missionary career path was consistent with the Medburys' religious convictions. Their Bible-based gender attitudes encouraged girls to be humble, pure, chaste, and self-sacrificing, and boys to build lucrative careers. Missionary work was acceptable for young women because it was assumed that it drew on their sensitive feminine qualities while also fulfilling their evangelical duty to spread the word of their faith.

Providence at the Advent of the 20th Century: Religion and Free Enterprise

It is important to explain the intricacies of Clara Thompson's religious foundational experience since these ideas saturated the air she breathed, shaping and coloring her experience and perspective. Thompson's family advocated living according to the principles of the Bible and attempted to bring others into the fold.

Historically, Thompson's hometown, Providence, welcomed dissenters of all kinds, offering shelter to people who were persecuted for their religious beliefs. It was also among the first cities in the nation to industrialize. By the 19th century, the city was one of America's leading ports of trade, and by the beginning of the 20th century, with its population of 175,597, the state capital, with its famous Market Square, was a center of commercial and social activity.

When Clara Thompson was born in 1893, religion, politics, and commerce were integral to the cultural life of Providence. The city's economy was at full throttle, led by burgeoning corporate firms including Brown and Sharpe, innovators in developing automatic machines and precision instruments; Gorham Manufacturing Company, the country's premier silverware manufacturer; and the American Screw Company, one of the nation's largest manufacturers of screws. Religious fundamentalism was increasingly shaping the circumstances of American life; as the city of Providence thrived economically, so too did evangelical Christianity, which had gained national prominence. The American historian George Marsden (2006) traces the rise of fundamentalism as a religious movement of American Christians who placed their confidence in the Bible. "Americans were proud of their own unique achievement since they had shown that the moral basis for national success could be maintained voluntarily without an officially established church" (p. 12).

The literary scholar Sacvan Bercovitch (2011) explains an important component of American history involving the Puritans' quest for religious freedom was the merging of a redemptive biblical story—the soul's journey to God, with commerce. He positions this spiritual quest within a secular search for economic opportunity and wealth in a new promised land. He explains how the Puritans raised the Protestant work ethic to the status of sainthood, then combined it into a community pact to achieve all that was possible—installing the idea as a national contract. It is argued that these two seemingly contradictory beliefs—one secular, the other religious—fueled an American drive toward self-realization, later refined and referred to as self-actualization (see Maslow, 1962), that advanced a cultural commitment to working to one's full potential. These are heady American history topics that are with apologies only highlighted here to provide some background on Clara Thompson's complex set of American values. Mitchell and Harris (2004) grappled with understanding "the Americanness of psychoanalysis" in the US in Thompson's era, the early and mid-20th century (p. 165) to comprehend its importance.

My aim is to provide a perspective on how some prevailing cultural influences shaped Clara Thompson. These complicated cultural influences go back to a New England that originally embraced the Puritan vision of John Winthrop, the first governor of the Massachusetts Bay Colony. Winthrop remarked that America should be an example to the world, the "shining city upon the hill." However, what these early New Englanders broadly proselytized was a skewed, settler-colonist view and a mindset of discrimination that still pervades American culture (Hannah-Jones, 2019). Slavery, brutality, and the exploitation of indigenous people existed in Massachusetts even before Winthrop arrived.

However, the Free Will Baptists,[2] Thompson's religious community, were strongly anti-slavery (Bryant, 2011). They worked to end slavery and supported the rights of indigenous people. They differed from the Southern Baptists in both their ideas about slavery and about salvation.[3]

American evangelicals had only the Bible as their doctrine, there was no central governing church. Instead, there were "churches" or "sects," of which the Free Will Baptists were one. "These denominations were the product of a combination of European churchly traditions, ethnic loyalties, pietism, sectarianism, and American free enterprise" (Marsden, 2006, p. 70). American evangelical Christians "enjoyed a remarkable consensus about the economic and moral laws that supported a sound economic system—that is, the prevailing free enterprise capitalism" (p. 13). They professed complete confidence in the Bible and were "preoccupied with the message of God's salvation of sinners through the death of Jesus Christ" (p. 3).

Scott Bryant (2011), an ordained Baptist minister, argues, "Where humility was a step toward salvation . . . the Free Baptist church empowered people to the extent that the divine initiative was lost and redemption became the product not of God's good pleasure but of human effort"

(p. 186). Noonday prayer meetings led by businessmen and bankers swept through the country in both the north and south, and "the Sabbath"—"a distinctive symbol of evangelical civilization" (p. 13)—became incorporated into American life.

Bryant describes the Free Will Baptists' break with Calvinism early in American religious history in New England:

> Their story was different: upcountry New England, rural origins; a subsection of the Great Awakening that morphed into a new theological tradition; a blended polity that resembled Wesleyan and Quaker ideas; in their context, a theologically liberating movement; a comprehensive program, national institutions, and recognition; conversancy with English General Baptist in a transatlantic community.
>
> (p. viii, Foreword)

Bryant sees the story of the Free Will Baptist movement as a uniquely American tale that has not yet been fully explored. As descendants of the General Baptists, this small evangelical denomination with a deep stronghold in New England made religion a way of life, not just a practice confined to Sunday mornings. Faith remained a condition for salvation; purity and self-sacrifice were mandated, especially for women; and the word of God as stated in the Bible was without error. The Free Will Baptists rejected predestination. They viewed predetermination as leading to a lack of self-effort and limiting social mobility. Instead they saw a choice to repent—the "free will" component—as a better option to salvation.

There were stark gender expectations guided by the perceived infallibility of the Bible that promoted the subordination of women: "Wives, be subject to your husband, as to the Lord. For the husband is the head of the wife as Christ is the head of the church" (Braude, 2000, p. 61). The family unit was the primary instrument of that subordination, in service of doing God's work and spreading the Christian faith.

The Inner Life of Adolescence

While all the biblical commandments were preached in the Thompson/Medbury household, the Fifth Commandment, "Honor thy father and thy mother," may have been particularly troublesome for young Clara

Thompson. Originally defined under a Puritan government, children were taught to honor all figures of authority. The Fifth Commandment was interpreted to include, "All our superiors, whether in Family, School, Church and Common-wealth" (Braude, 2000, p. 70). It was also the case that "[t]he wife's authority equaled her husband's as a parent of children" (p. 75). Thompson's mother's life, like that of many of her friends, would have revolved around the Free Will Baptist community. As a Sunday school teacher, she would have stressed the evangelical ideal of womanhood, which demanded self-sacrifice and chastity. And, her mother was likely judged by her community for how well her daughter adhered to the rules, which may in part explain why she was such a strict enforcer.

Clara Thompson left no written record or diary as an adolescent to help us better understand how the small and large events in her life played out and, how she felt about them; however, we do have an undated handwritten poem that speaks to her budding sexuality.

Hand-written Poem by Clara Mabel Thompson (Date Unknown)

One day, Willie, a little girl did meet
She asked him a question, he took a seat.
Then everyone began to say,
So you <u>have a fellow</u> today.
Then everyone began to brush
Poor Mabel's feeling and made her blush
Then she said to Willie
What <u>makes them act</u> so silly
Said Willie, "What have we done,
To let them have such fun.
Then went she from him very . . .
And wishing <u>that she</u> had been bad
And had let him know
That it was not all for show,
That she really cared for him
Though <u>he did not care</u> a thing
At first she did not really care

With him her lot to share,
But many times she'd quickly say
Why not <u>love him</u> anyway.
They think I do at least
I'm tired of shamming like a beast.

Then came an invitation while,
~~Cape Cod~~ <u>Which made poor Mabel</u> happy quite
Hatteras For t'was from Della, Willie's sis
Who said ~~she~~ I must not miss
Such an opportunity
To <u>come and take</u> some tea
With Willie and the rest,
And do her very best,
To get a seat by him,
And <u>then how</u> ~~we~~ <u>they</u> did skim
Over the forfeit time
Without one kiss in fine
Although one time they tried
And in ~~the closet~~ tried
And tried to make them ~~us~~ kiss
But they ~~we~~ tried hard to miss.
And later Willie's father strong
Said, "~~What has gone~~ so very wrong
Carl replied, "Oh that's Bill's girl
And we've got her in a whirl Till she don't know where she is
And <u>wishes we'd mind</u> our biss"

Said Wille's father looking straight
At those brown eyes as true as fate
"Well she looks like a nice little girl,
Pretty enough to be Bill's pearl.
If she, he cares to choose
I'm sure he will not loose."
And she did redder grow,
'Till her <u>face was in a</u> bright glow.
But I'm afraid it cannot be

For Willie to care for me,
And so I tell you this sad, sad tale,
That love on one side will surly fail,
If tisn't the other side too
For I am Mabel.

The undated poem, possibly written during her adolescent years, suggests her attraction to a boy and the shaming she experienced around her first kiss. The expression of affection became a central issue in her psychoanalytic treatment with Sándor Ferenczi. Thompson's autobiographical sounding clinical case studies provide a window into the feelings she possibly experienced as that young girl. In "Childhood" (Thompson, 1964b), Thompson expressed her understanding of how parental attitudes around gender shape children's behavior.

> When a child is born, all too frequently a boy or a girl is hopefully awaited. If the child turns out to be the "wrong" sex the parents are markedly disappointed . . . whatever the prenatal attitude toward the sex of the child, from birth on the actual sex subtly influences the reactions of the significant adults toward the baby.
>
> (Thompson, 1964b, p. 295)

Elizabeth Capelle (1993) points us to Thompson's description in "Psychopathology of Adolescence" (Thompson, 1964c)[4] as another source of biographical information about Thompson's experiences as an adolescent and her own rude awakening:

> So the girl who may have led a life of comparative freedom up to the beginning of adolescence, suddenly finds her goings and comings a matter of close supervision. The mother may talk to her vaguely about "bad boys," about the general lack of self-control of the male, or the daughter may be given lofty sentiments about her duty in uplifting boys and keeping them moral. At any rate, the upshot of the matter is that one must not be touched by a boy, and a kiss is a very serious matter. A girl may even worry over being ruined, being "damaged goods," if such a liberty is permitted. Girls who prior to adolescence have already fallen unduly under the sway of such a mother early

become discouraged in their tentative efforts toward normal development. They cannot go out with boys without transgressing their standards—it therefore becomes easier to keep away from boys and to take
refuge in the preadolescent relationship with girl friends.

(Thompson, 1964c, p. 310)

Thompson's (1959) "An Introduction to Minor Maladjustments" further
echoes these autobiographical sounding reflections on the constraints
imposed by her religion on adolescent girlhood.

A young girl blossoming into adolescence was presented with a problem which seemed to change her whole way of life from one of outgoing friendliness and popularity to one of introversion and withdrawal.
She had been brought up under the influence of a Protestant sect which
taught the necessity of denial of the pleasures of the flesh.

(p. 241–242)

Following Thompson's presentation of the "patient" she notes that the
girl's companions in childhood had all shared similar backgrounds, such
that these restrictions had not particularly affected her—"until she reached
the age when sex became a factor in relationships" (p. 242):

In high school, she encountered, for the first time, another cultural
group, but she still continued to be popular with boys and girls until
she came to the first high-school dance.
    She had been taught that dancing was wicked, and she had never
questioned this teaching. She had not been allowed to take dancing
lessons, and she had not been fully aware of how this made her different from others until she went to the party. At the dance, her friends
came and asked for dances, and suddenly she found that she was all
wrong—different. She had to say, "I don't know how to dance," and
"My parents don't want me to dance." That evening, she experienced
with horror, the feeling that she was a wallflower, and from that day
she could not regain her old self-confidence.

(p. 242)

Thompson explains that the profound and sudden loss of confidence was
not because her friends had dropped her or because she felt she could

no longer interest them and so withdrew from her peers. Nor was it the result of that one evening being ruined. Rather, she envisioned a future that would be deprived of the joys shared with her peers. This was one of her first decision points.

> Before she would be able again to feel that she belonged, she would have to think through her convictions about attitudes she had accepted without question up to that point.

(p. 242)

Crosscurrents: The Women's Missionary Society and the Women's Suffragist Movement

Thompson's values were formed within her New England religious community, where service to others, and to God, was imposed by the leaders of the Free Will Baptist Church. Service to God was also important to the Free Baptist Women's Missionary Society, to which her mother belonged. As Capelle (1993) writes,

> The Free [Will] Baptist women, like the women of other denominations, had taken on themselves the task of recruiting and supporting single women missionaries—particularly medical missionaries—in the belief that the secluded women of India could be reached only by women, and that the wives of the male missionaries, with their family responsibilities, had little time or energy for the task.

(p. 141)

Between 1873 and 1921, the Women's Missionary Society was an active, well-run organization that sent young women to India, China, and other countries to convert people to Christianity. Its members raised money, taught Sunday school, and spread the word of Christ. Their motto sums up their mission:

> And this is your commission
> O women, saved by grace,
> To tell of Christ arisen

To all the human race.
(Free Baptist Woman's
Missionary Society,
1873–1921 (1980), p. 13)

Like other evangelicals, the Free Will Baptists had a mission for saving souls.

> Capelle (1993) explains that as a Free Baptist woman, "one could be, the evangelist to one's family as Mrs. Thompson seems to have been; one could take up Sunday school teaching or benevolent work, as women increasingly did . . . ; or one could become a foreign missionary, as the young Clara Thompson had planned to do."
>
> (p. 139–140)

Becoming a missionary was viewed as the highest form of benevolent work. The young Thompson likely saw a path independent of her mother's choice when she announced her intension to become a medical missionary. Medical missionaries performed a combination of social work and community service with an emphasis on physical and spiritual healing. However, in addition to being a healer of physical disease and a saver of souls, there were rigid social requirements, including a professed dedication to a life of self-sacrifice and self-denial. Elizabeth Capelle notes that "Women missionaries were required to be single—if they married, they resigned their positions." As Capelle points out, "part of their 'mission' was to carry restrictive standards of sexual morality to the heathen" (1993, p. 148). Social and evangelical work went hand in hand for medical missionaries. To become a missionary was a calling to service.

When 15-year-old Clara Thompson declared her intention to become a medical missionary, she was most likely captured by the romantic thought that she could be part of a larger effort to relieve the suffering of the distressed. She was only vaguely aware that choosing to become a missionary meant renouncing any plans for marriage or children, since women missionaries were required to dedicate their lives to the denial of pleasure and accept asceticism. Thompson eventually became torn between a conflicting desire for a life of love and adventure and the missionary's life of virtuous deprivation and self-denial. She chafed at the tension between her mother's strong ideals and the budding sense of her own desires. As she expressed it in her interview for the Freud Archives (1952),

> I had a great difficulty with a rigid mother, who was very religious and very—she was really a very frightened person but she covered it up with this controlling rigidity; "You must do this and you mustn't do that."

An unnamed friend affirmed this view of Thompson's mother, describing her as "a dominating personality, very religious—with firmly set notions of what constituted proper behavior for a Christian young woman" (Capelle, 1993, p. 145).

The Other Cultural Influence

Aside from religion, the other cultural force that actively shaped Clara Thompson's life was a robust women's movement fighting for suffrage and broader social, civil, religious, and educational rights for women. In July of 1848, the Seneca Falls Convention had issued a declaration of sentiments calling on women to fight for women's constitutional right to equality, including being able to vote, hold property, and obtain an education.

While these early feminists focused on securing the right to vote, the women's movement increasingly came to include those who sought more than suffrage. Their goals encompassed sexual emancipation, economic independence through education, self-fulfillment through work, and a general end to sex stereotyping. The Rhode Island Women's Suffrage Association actively fought for the rights of women despite meeting setbacks.[5] In Thompson's hometown of Providence, women actively began petitioning for access to higher education. In 1891 a local resident, a teacher, and educational reformer Sarah Doyle, successfully led a campaign to admit women to Brown University, and established Pembroke College, the women's college at Brown. By 1893, the year of Thompson's birth, the women's movement had begun to open higher education, allowing women to enter the professions.[6] Indeed, Thompson would directly benefit from these hard-won changes; she attended college and went on to complete medical school in 1920, joining the ranks of women physicians in the United States—at that time there were around 10% in cities like Boston.[7]

The conflict between her Baptist religion and her desire for self-realization, so significant for the young Thompson, was more broadly reflected in the intersection of women's rights and women's religious groups—the two powerful social forces that deeply informed her developing ethos. Those strange bedfellows both sought to assert the rights of women, demanding of the individual that she live a life of excellence based on actualizing her human potential. The goals of the women's movement—"universal suffrage and civil rights [as] key components of America's identity as a democratic nation" (Braude, 1989, p. 12)—in many ways dovetailed with those of the progressive wing of the Women's Missionary Society. What is left unsaid is that they were white privileged Americans. Helen Barrett Montgomery, a "preeminent figure in the interdenominational women's missionary movement," preached that the "gospel is the most tremendous engine of democracy . . . destined to break in pieces all castes, privileges, and oppressions . . . perhaps the last caste to be destroyed will be that of sex" (Capelle, 1993, p. 203).

"Woman's work for woman" became a slogan of the women's missionary movement. Indeed, the women who served as medical missionaries believed that they were both saving the souls of heathens and uplifting them from "the abject position prescribed for women by pagan religions" (Capelle, 1993, p. 142). From Capelle (1993) we learn that Helen Barrett Montgomery argued for uplifting Christian women and endorsed separate missionary organizations for women through the assertion that "the opportunity for self-expression and the development that comes through responsibility are as necessary to women as to men" (p. 203). For these very reasons, some members within the Baptist women's community were less enthusiastic about the women's missionary movement and questioned its motives. Was it truly a vehicle for women to help put their special abilities of self-sacrifice and self-denial to good Christian use or was it a vehicle for women to argue for equality using missionary work as a front?

As women's roles in society became a theme in the late 19th and early 20th centuries, two primary perspectives developed: one that focused on the value of women's "essential qualities," the other focused largely on women's equality. The first view, grounded primarily in Europe, held that women had a special duty to use what were seen as inherent qualities and apply them beyond the bounds of the home. This view held that women's "special nature," including maternal functions, be regarded as equal in value to men's capacities and occupations. In contrast, a "different but equal" view claimed that women were equal to men and had rights to freedom and self-development, hard stop. Established primarily in the United States, this idea of equality maintained that women held no essential differences from men and, as such, deserved all the rights and opportunities of men.

This deep dive into the religious beliefs of the Free Baptist community is important because these are the beliefs that influenced Clara Thompson's young life. She broke with her religion in college. There are no glimmerings of spirituality in her essays but she did retain a set of values that spoke to a moral compass of her own, to be fair, non-judgmental, honest, simple, and forthright. She commented to a friend, "I could not be complicated if I tried" (Green, 1964, p. 375), suggesting that being forthright was part of her DNA. Her humility ran deep. It could also be heard as an "American superficiality" rooted in a "national character" (Layton, 2004, p. 236) or in Cushman's (1996) sense as part of the language of the "dominant culture" of New England (p. 297). Clara Thompson was a liberal, white, privileged American woman. The tools to unpack her white privilege were decades away and out of reach for her. In college, she grew increasingly unhappy as the gulf between the religious culture of her early life and her aspirations about her future life grew wider.

Pembroke College, Class of 1916

In 1912, nineteen-year-old Clara Thompson matriculated at nearby Pembroke College founded in 1891 as the women's college of Brown University. In view of her high school achievements, Thompson could have had her pick of the top women's colleges in the country—Wellesley, Smith, or Radcliffe. But she chose to apply locally to Pembroke. As a local "commuting student," she lived at home. She was a good student and focused on learning. Her major in premedical studies was acceptable to her mother because it fit the medical missionary path. But she also took courses on the English Bible, 19th-century literature, philosophy, and sociology. A friend recalls that she and Thompson "frequently had lunch together and Clara would talk eagerly and excitedly about what she was learning in science" (Green, 1964, p. 350). During her senior year, due to her outstanding academic achievement, she was elected to Phi Beta Kappa and Sigma Xi.

The history of Pembroke College is a part of the history of women's equality. Pembroke was founded after a young woman had applied to then all-male

Brown University and was rejected. The governing committee deliberated for years on the issue of whether to admit women before deciding to create an adjunctive women's college while maintaining Brown as an all-men's institution. The women's college began as Pembroke Hall, named after its principal building, and was not officially named Pembroke College in Brown University until 1928. Like other elite institutions at that time, such as Columbia University/Barnard College and Harvard University/Radcliffe College, Pembroke provided women with a first-rate college education. Brown University did not become completely co-educational until 1971.

The first Pembroke classes were held at a boy's grammar school; the young women had to arrive at the school at 2 o'clock, after the male students were dismissed. Since the building had no electricity, the women worked until the light faded, which in the winter was at 5 pm. Sarah Doyle, a Providence native known as an American educator and reformer of women's education, formed the Rhode Island Society for the Collegiate Education of Women and raised $75,000 to build the first permanent building for Pembroke's students. During the years 1912 to 1916 when Thompson was in attendance, she did not take classes in the new Pembroke College building.

While Thompson was enrolled at Pembroke, "Women [comprised] about one quarter of the undergraduate student body" of Brown University (Capelle, 1993, p. 158). The Pembroke buildings were located several blocks from campus, a more than metaphoric separation of the women's college from the men's. The women were continually aware of their difference in status. Drawing closely on Capelle's (1993) discussion we learn that at Pembroke/Brown University, "the message to women students was mixed" (p. 171). The female students were aware that the school's teaching faculty and researchers were mostly male and that specializations in research were closed to them . . .

> not only did the Women's College suffer from second-class status within the university, but while formally receiving the same education as the male students, women received mixed messages about their seriousness as students and the purpose of their education.
>
> (p. 158)

The Pembroke Center Oral History Project at Brown University provides a collection of remembrances that give further voice to the various ways that

Thompson's classmates, and by extension Thompson herself, experienced Pembroke and how those experiences influenced their lives. Recurring themes within these women's stories during the period in which Thompson was enrolled include their treatment as lower-status students than their male counterparts at Brown, the strict rules of dress and comportment, and the all-work-and-no-fun attitude of the college leadership. These remembrances also express appreciation—for Pembroke's academic excellence. They enjoyed the opportunity to be immersed in an atmosphere of intellectual stimulation and development, and the *esprit de corps* of the women students. They appreciated the opportunity, and encouragement, to participate in athletics and physical exercise. Indeed, the holdings of the Pembroke Oral History Project paint a complex and sometimes conflicted picture of college life for these young women in the first decades of the 20th century.

In describing her first-year experience living in the Pembroke dormitory, Marjorie Phillips Wood (Burroughs, n.d.), Class of 1911, recalls how the electric car ran past her house in Taunton and brought her to campus in an hour. The trip was thought to be too much, so she lived in what was then the dormitory at Slater Memorial Homestead on Benefit Street. She recalls that about 15 girls lived in the dorm and that they all climbed the steep hill up to Pembroke Hall every morning. Wood remembers the rigid dress code at Pembroke along with other restrictions, noting that women students were not allowed to go to the John Hay Library without "our hat and gloves on." In fact, the students created a song: "Wear your gloves and veil and hat, always do remember that; because you are a Pembroke girl."

Lida Shaw King, an American classics scholar, was the college dean. A graduate of both Vassar College (1890) and an early graduate of Pembroke/Brown University (1894), King also was the first woman allowed to attend the American School of Classical Studies at Athens, Greece, founded in 1881. Following her appointment as Dean, she created a program to better understand the issues of the Pembroke College students. King established lectures to orient new students to the school and sponsored discussions with special invited speakers. She was successful in broadening the composition of the student body, appealing to students from outside the state of Rhode Island. She also held "puritanical" views on correct "associations" between men and women at the college (Hawk, 1967, p. 113).

Gladys Paine (Johnson, 1986), Class of 1913, recounts that during fresh-
man year, everyone had Latin classes taught by Dean King:

> She was very strict. We were a little scared of her, but she was an excel-
> lent Dean and I think she impressed me very favorably. Her mind was
> so keen and—of course, they always gave little homilies at chapel . . .
> she always had something worthwhile to say.

Wood describes Dean King as "tall and slender, and she had lovely curly
hair—very wavy. And quite classy features. A very nice nose, and eyes
and uh, a very good looking woman, but she did inspire awe. I think," adds
(Burroughs, n.d.). Students also recalled how Dean King would give ser-
mons in the chapel emphasizing the importance of their dress and general
appearance. King's views on dress and appropriate behavior for women
surely had an impact on Clara Thompson, who attended her compulsory
chapel services four mornings a week. This becomes important later to
counter accusations around issues of hygiene and appearance that emerge
in the Clinical Diary (see chapter 4).

Ruth Dorothea (Peterson, n.d.), Class of 1919, elaborated on what she
thought were "stirrings" among the parents of her generation regarding
what they wanted for their daughters—a rigorous college education—but
that left Pembroke students feeling very pressured:

> Too much studying, too much—everything was very restricted . . .
> one had to stick to the courses to the time of lectures, which were 50
> minutes, and there was so much preparation, that after your classes
> were over, it was to the John Hay library, or another library . . . And
> everybody was bent on business. There was none of this meeting and
> getting all the gossip and having all the merriments, you know?

Peterson goes on to describe the stark gender differences between Pembroke and Brown students' experiences this way:

> It was quite different then. It was really, while we did have a Brown
> University degree, classes were kept very, very separate, and profes-
> sors came to Pembroke to give their courses. The students did not go
> to the hill[8] with few exceptions. We did not have a laboratory, there-
> fore all laboratory work had to be done on the hill.

Being on the basketball team in college was the happiest time of all, Peterson recalls; her father would say "she was the best boy he had."

One might assume that this level of physical activity was unusual for the young girls in Providence at this point in time, but it was not. In fact, it was socially acceptable for them to achieve a sense of body competence and to enjoy the competition of athletic sports; In preadolescence, young women were encouraged to participate in sports, competitive and agentic behavior was acceptable. At Pembroke, these activities continued. But as Thompson later understood, the imposition of cultural restrictions ultimately presented a conflict for women leading to feelings of shame, losses of freedom and equality with boys, and the right to be aggressive. (see Thompson, 1947).

One student, Marguerite (Appleton, n.d.), Class of 1914, pointed out that "not all students were pre-med at Pembroke but they were all on the basketball teams, bowling teams, and other sport and dancing events." Another student, Alita Bosworth Cameron (Cameron & Sherman, n.d.), Class of 1914, said, "We really tried to know everybody in the class and of course with only 50 you could." Rowena Sherman (Cameron & Sherman, n.d.), graduated from Classical High School in the class of 1914, so conceivably she and Thompson would have known each other. Like Thompson, Sherman lived at home and noted the savings in dormitory costs and the fact that eighty percent of the students lived at home. Sherman recounted that her classmates came from various places but that "most of us were Providence girls." She explained how Pembroke students had a choice of languages but that they all "had to take Latin." She also remarked that few class members went into the "German division." Thompson learned only enough German to meet the requirement for entry to Johns Hopkins, she never took the class at Pembroke.

Thompson was a member of the Question Club—a club whose members were presented with phrases and asked to come up with meaningless answers. That may explain her curious answer in her college yearbook to the question, Future plans?—"to murder people in the most refined way possible" (Green, 1964, p. 351).

Pembroke was a place of intellectual rigor and challenge for all students. She was introduced to a cultural group different from the religious community of her childhood. In this academic world, science, discovery, and self-realization were what mattered with an emphasis on improving the collective good. As Walter Goodnow Everett (1918), one of Thompson's teachers at Pembroke/Brown, argues in his published lectures to undergraduates, "All human activities, it is shown, are judged to be good or bad, better or worse, according to the contribution which they are thought to make to the worth of human life as a whole" (pp. v-vi).

The academics at Pembroke/Brown underscored that self-realization encouraged "the free man (sic)" to develop all his capacities, to become a master of himself by realizing a common good that was the rational basis of the social order. The fact that "women" were not included in the text was no accident. The double message of blatant sexism and social realities did not preclude Pembroke from also challenging its women students and encouraging them toward self-realization.

The English literature course taught by Lindsay Todd Damon was one such example.[9] He was an animated lecturer who stirred a passion for learning in his students. The Pembroke Oral History Project, Brown University, describes his class as follows:

> Damon loved to read from Swinburne and it wouldn't take him long to warm up to his task. His face would get red, his white hair would fly, and he would roll out those lines like an actor on a stage. Sometimes right in the middle of a reading the students would catch the fever of the moment and show their appreciation by stamping their feet in unison until one would think the old floor was going to go crashing down.
>
> (Pembroke Oral History
> Project, Brown University)[10]

As one female student put it, "to me he was the man who pulled the foundations out from under us and sent us searching" (Green, 1964, p. 350). Capelle (1993) writes that Damon promoted

> a skepticism about received ideas, [but] he was at one with other American humanists of the era in rejecting the pessimistic strain of European culture. He retained an earnest concern with morality and ethics, endorsing, as he once wrote, "belief in the worth of 'Gooddeeds,' and a . . . vital sense of personal responsibility—to God or the universe, as one's own theology dictates."
>
> (Capelle, 1993, p. 153)

Capelle (1993) quotes a student who stated that Damon taught them "to think for themselves, not to take [ideas] 'off the counter' as he called it" (pp. 152–153).

In college, Thompson began to realize she had been hiding her real feelings for quite some time. She learned to imagine a different way of being.

As a youngster, Thompson appeared compliant on the surface, but her obedience was only a way to placate others, particularly her mother. She hid her real feelings to keep the peace.[11]

The demand from her mother's side of the family to be conforming, meek, and humble openly collided with the call from the likes of Damon and other emancipatory Pembroke influences to open her mind and imagination in forging a future for herself. It was in Damon's course that Thompson read *The Mill on the Floss* by George Eliot (1860) and became enthralled with the central character, Maggie, with whom she identified. A classmate quoted in Green (1964) describes:

> Clara identified herself with the character "Maggie," and for years signed herself so in our correspondence, and I so addressed her. She seemed to have very few friends outside her field of science, perhaps because at the time most of the Women's College was local, and Clara was not the New England type . . . She was, moreover, far beyond us in intellect. The only college activity I remember her participating in was debate, in which hardly any one could stand up to her.
>
> (Green, 351)

As Capelle sees it, "Thompson's identification with Maggie Tulliver reveals her own continuing struggle with the conflict between self-sacrificing devotion to duty—religious and familial or social"—and a "wider life" (p. 168). Maggie abandons her wish for happiness and adopts a selfless existence. "She pities the unfortunate and unhappy, wanting to give them what she herself has yearned for and not received" (Capelle, p. 168).

This was a pivotal time in Clara Thompson's life. After reading *The Mill on the Floss*, she stopped attending church services and dropped the name Mabel. For a time she used the name Maggie but then reclaimed her given name Clara. After a long painful struggle, she distanced herself from her mother. That rupture lasted nearly twenty years.

Thompson began to develop a nuanced awareness of how conflicting cultural norms and attitudes—especially around gender and religion—functioned in what she refers to in her later work as "the great melting pot of American life" (Thompson, 1959, p. 242). She also said that people often come into conflict with "their earlier cultural patterns," explaining: "This has been especially dramatically shown in the rapid movement of the last fifty years toward the 'emancipation' of women" (Thompson, 1959, p. 242). Here Thompson offers a cultural explanation as the cause of distress, rather than attributing it to individual pathology or to women's inherent nature. She goes on to explain that conflicting cultural attitudes cause internal confusion, arguing that this confusion should not be considered an emotional disturbance because it develops from positive strengths that are seeking growth in new ways of living. Thompson sees the individual, and perhaps her younger self, as struggling to shake free of restrictive cultural directives—a reasonable and productive inclination, and not an individual personality problem.

Thompson's interests never developed in the direction "of the traditional American ideal" meaning as a wife and mother (Green, 1964, p. 205). She struggled to free herself of cultural directives as one of her classmates' descriptions reveals.

> Until Mr. Damon's course, Clara was preparing to be a medical mis-sionary. We dutifully went to the Baptist Church on Sunday, but at night Clara would pour her heart out, trying to express her unsatisfied longings and frustrations. I was quite unprepared for what she seemed to expect of me in support and inspiration, and I was afraid of her intensity, never having known it in any one before, and in few since . . . After our second year we had no further contact in the classroom since she was taking advanced courses in science and I language and history. She was living at home and I in the one dormitory the Women's College then had.
>
> (Green, 1964, p. 351)

Thompson's growing dissatisfaction with, and ultimate rejection of, her decision to become a medical missionary shook her foundation. She strug-gled with her earlier wish to dedicate her life to the service of others and her growing interest in science and self-discovery. The missionary move-ment, at least in fantasy, had offered a way to remain true to her family's values, maintaining a respected place in the world of her mother. Now her growing goal was to achieve a fuller, more autonomous life for herself. She wanted to improve the lives of others, not save their souls.

Other recollections of peers from her Pembroke years draw a complicated picture of a young woman in conflict. For example, a friend recalled Thompson visiting her at her family's home.

> She was so quiet and seemed to get a warm pleasure—you could feel it—out of our comfortable atmosphere. I am sure no one said or did anything of note, and all I can remember is that we could meet on a non-demanding level of friendliness. I was in no class with her and never thought of her brilliance; just that she was such a good person.
>
> (Green, 1964, p. 350)

This quality of interpersonal warmth endured throughout her life.

Throughout college, Thompson remained intellectually hungry and academically successful but unhappy. The academic accolades she received did not change her sense of loneliness and the embittered feelings that had surfaced as she entered adolescence and felt her family's disapproval. The year Thompson graduated from Pembroke, the editors of the 1916 yearbook printed a blurb under each photograph. Thompson's reads: "Blessed with a knowledge both of book and humankind." The editors also had submitted a list of questions to the graduating students; as noted before, Thompson's future plans were—"to murder people in the most refined way possible." Her chief virtues—"supreme faith in myself"; dislikes—"sleep"; likes—"a lot of interesting things"; fads—"being pious and studious"; ambitions—"to succeed in my fads and overcome my virtues."

> (Green, 1964, p. 351)

During her time at Pembroke, Thompson had developed a clearer sense of who she was and what she wanted, she seemed to possess a fine sense of humor. The line "to murder people in the most refined way possible"[12] still gives us pause. Does this "joke" reveal something dark about Thompson's personality? Could the line speak to her fear of the awesome responsibility of becoming a physician—that to make a mistake might result in someone's death?

Ferenczi said he saw something of himself in Thompson. He questioned if efforts to help people might conceal darker motives. To Shapiro (1993) the line suggests an underlying "rage and hostility," citing emotions Ferenczi thought were beneath Thompson's conventional demeanor (p. 165).

Thompson graduated from Pembroke with honors in biology, chemistry, romance languages, and literature. Her academic successes led to her receiving high honors.[13] By the time of graduation, she had abandoned her initial plan to become a medical missionary in favor of studying medicine. She broke off communication with her rigidly religious mother and rejected a proposal of marriage that would have restricted her desire to establish an independent life.[14] She was stepping outside of the culture.

The Difficult Road Ahead

Two letters[15] precede her actual application to medical school. They illustrate her tenacity and commitment to her goal of becoming a physician. In the first, written on January 14, 1915, while she was still a junior at Pembroke, she anticipates a potential problem with her application:

> Dear Sir: I am looking over your requirements for admission to medical school and find that I shall have some difficulty in fulfilling the requirements because our college courses do not exactly fit. I am a student at Brown University and I shall be graduated in June 1916 . . . I have another year in which to get the requirements which I shall need. I am particularly troubled over the requirements in chemistry and physics . . . What do you think would be best for me to do? My professor in chemistry says that he is willing to make some special arrangements for me in laboratory work . . . I do not wish to take qualitative analysis if there is any other way in which I can get those four laboratory hours because it will mean more extra work than I ought to carry next year . . . There is only one other difficulty. I have not studied German in any school. I have started to study it by myself. I have thought that being able to read it is of more importance than the grammar and I have consequently paid no more attention than was absolutely necessary to grammar. I presume that I shall have to take an examination in German . . . ? Will the study of it as I have described be sufficient? If you will straighten out these matters for me I shall be very much obliged to you.
>
> Sincerely, Clara M. Thompson.
>
> (Thompson, 1915a)

Thompson was not about overburden herself as she explains as someone possessed of self-awareness. The ability to state her needs directly would be with her all of her life.[16]

During her senior year at college, Thompson sent a follow-up letter to Johns Hopkins on September 28, 1915, (Thompson, 1915b). This time she was writing to say that she had fulfilled all the requirements except for one—she had taken only a half-year of German but intended to get additional experience over the winter. Her organic chemistry text was written in German so she anticipated that would sharpen her skills in the language. Her application to medical school, dated April 20, 1916, included a recommendation from Dean Linda Shaw King.

Where Thompson's early aspirational career to become a medical missionary had offered the possibility of adventure and personal achievement,[17] going to medical school to become a physician was an outright act of rebellion. Later in life she asserted, "the child may rebel, but in his rebellion, he is unhappy and insecure," noting that "the basic mores of a particular culture are written into the developing personality" (Thompson, 1958, p. 8). In no small part through her own early experiences, Thompson came to believe that character was deeply influenced by culture.

After rejecting the path her mother wished for her, she would never again turn her interests toward helping people develop their relationship to God. Instead, she devoted herself to curing the sick. She ascribed to the belief that it was an individual's purpose to develop their talents through their personal growth and independence. Over time, her psychosocial/interpersonal perspective would serve to transform her childhood zeal for changing lives through belief in God into a zeal for changing lives through the self-discovery process of psychoanalysis. Not surprisingly, Erich Fromm (1964, *Foreword*, p. v) said that Thompson was one of the most self-actualized people he knew. Harry Stack Sullivan seems to have felt the same way—Perry (1982) reports that "Sullivan considered Thompson an important exception to his theory that in this society all of us are poor caricatures of what we might have been; Thompson had lived up to all her potentialities, according to Sullivan" (p. 207).[18]

Clara Thompson fits the picture of one of the rare mavericks whose life experiences made her a rebel rather than a conformist. During her foundational years, she establish a sense of honesty and integrity and a pragmatic approach to the world which she eventually brought to her perspective on psychoanalysis. Long before meeting Ferenczi, her ideas about respect and fairness were central to how she dealt with others. While she abandoned religion because of its restrictions and prohibitions, Thompson did not forsake the mission to bring about a kinder world. A peaceful mind or psyche was an objective in meeting that goal. The next phase of her life would usher in an opportunity to affirm those ideals with a new group of friends and colleagues whose notions of the good life matched her own.

> "As she said, "In important ways, the meaning of each stage of life is dependent on what happened in the preceding stages.""
>
> Thompson (1964a, p. 335)

She said that children who identify with their parents out of fear find it difficult, if not impossible, to achieve a necessary critical distance from their parents' attitudes. She describes a situation with a patient that sounds very close to her own experience. She says, "a young girl blossoming into adolescence was presented with a problem which seemed to change her whole way of life from one of outgoing friendliness and popularity to one of introversion and withdrawal" (Thompson, 1959, p. 241). This clinical example offers a glimpse into her feelings as an adolescent. She discusses a patient who was brought up under the influence of a Protestant sect, "which taught the necessity of denial of the pleasures of the flesh":

> In childhood, this had not particularly affected her, because her companions had similar backgrounds. She was perhaps more serious minded than some of her playmates, but she was good at sports and a popular leader until she reached the age when sex becomes a factor in relationships.
>
> (p. 242)

As a clinician, she perhaps extrapolates her own early experience into an understanding of how minor maladjustments in life can develop as she reasons how a "subcultural attitude" can make a person an outcast. Her individual development may have influenced how came to understand the aim of clinical psychoanalysis.

Thompson characteristically was not threatened or afraid of ambiguity or change; instead, she grew comfortable with it and sought it out. She became a standard-bearer of the American feminist point of view and an advocate of similar values in her approach to psychoanalysis. Ultimately, Thompson tried to integrate the values of fairness and honesty from her early religious training with the process of self-discovery and personal autonomy.

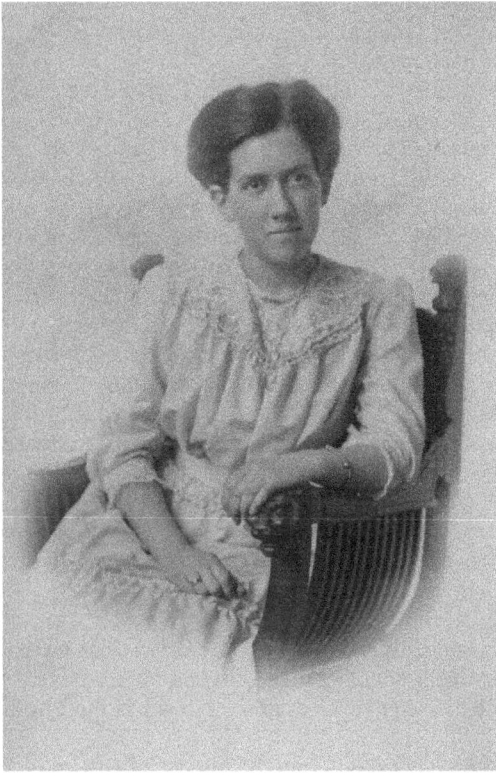

Figure 2.1 Clara Thompson at the time of her graduation from high school; ca. 1912–1916. Reprinted with permission, © William Alanson White Institute.

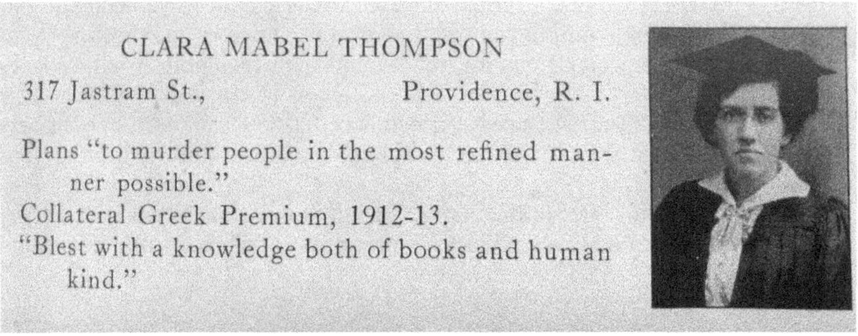

CLARA MABEL THOMPSON

317 Jastram St.,   Providence, R. I.

Plans "to murder people in the most refined man-
    ner possible."
Collateral Greek Premium, 1912-13.
"Blest with a knowledge both of books and human
    kind."

Figure 2.2 Clara Thompson in her graduation yearbook. Reprinted with permission, © William Alanson White Institute.

Notes

1 Thompson's last will indicates her mother's name was "Medbury," not "Medberry," as other sources report.
2 After 1841, The Freewill Baptists of New England were called the Free Baptists. They were the most successful break with the Calvinists Baptist camp in early American religious history (Bryant, 2011).
3 Free Will Baptists believed that salvation was not guaranteed; Baptists felt that once a person accepts salvation they were saved forever.
4 Thompson told Perry (1982) she wrote this chapter anonymously for Sullivan's book *Personal Psychopathology* (1965).
5 The Rhode Island Union of Colored Women's Clubs became the largest women's group to endorse women's suffrage in the state in 1913.
6 The ratio of (white) male to female undergraduates in the United States was about equal from 1900 to 1930 (Goldin et al., 2006). The gender imbalance in college attendance began in the 1930s and continued to grow following WWII. But professional women at the turn of the century were scarce. Between 1870 and 1930, the percentage of women in the professions slowly increased from 5% of all employed women in 1870 to 14% in 1930 (see Parker, 2015). These gains were happening despite the fact that some colleges restricted women's access to higher education by enforcing quotas that limited the number of women qualified for the professions.
7 Those numbers declined in 1940.
8 The "hill" was where the Brown University buildings were located.
9 Damon, a Harvard graduate, taught English at Brown and at the University of Chicago and subsequently became the head of the English Department at Brown.
10 Martha Mitchell's (1993) work on the history of Brown University, *Encyclopedia Brunoniana*. Mitchell, M. (1993). "Damon, Lindsay Todd." Encyclopedia Brunoniana, Brown University Library.
11 Later as a psychoanalyst, she drew from her early experiences to explicate how compliance can be used as a defensive operation that provides short-term relief from anxiety but long-term character problems. In her 1931 essay, " 'Dutiful Child': Resistance," she discusses the ways accommodation to the other—compliance can function to suppress real feelings that become lost from conscious awareness and then reemerge in analysis as resistance.
12 At Pembroke all heads of clubs were members of the Question Club. Members devised nonsensical lines. This may explain the curious line "to murder people . . ."
13 Grace Hawk (1967) traced the first seventy-five years of Pembroke College. In discussing the many accomplished women who graduated from the college she notes that, "Clara Thompson'16 practiced and wrote on psychoanalysis" (p. 95).
14 As an undergraduate, Thompson had dated a young man, a major in the United States medical corps. He wanted to marry her; however, his marriage proposal was contingent on her giving up her plans for a career in medicine.

15 The Alan Mason Chesney Medical Archives of the Johns Hopkins Medical Institution contains the letters related to Thompson's application to its Medical Department.
16 Thompson never achieved proficiency in German.
17 Thompson's father had stood in some ways apart from her mother, and it was his ambition that dominated his life, not religion.
18 Perry considered Sullivan's remark harsh and understood it as Sullivan's wanting to dampen any hopes Thompson may have had about his availability for a romantic relationship. We cannot know if that was Perry's fantasy or Sullivan's.

References

Appleton, M. (n.d.). *Marguerite Appleton, class of 1914*. [Audio file]. Pembroke Center Oral History Project. Brown University. www.brown.edu/initiatives/pembroke-oral-histories/interview/marguerite-appleton-class-1914

Bercovitch, S. (2011). *The Puritan origins of the American self*. Yale University Press.

Braude, A. (1989). *Radical spirits: Spiritualism and women's rights in nineteenth-century America*. Beacon Press.

Braude, A. (2000). *Sisters and saints: Women and American religion*. Oxford University Press.

Bryant, S. (2011). *The awakening of the Freewill Baptists: Benjamin Randall and the founding of an American religious tradition*. Mercer University Press.

Burroughs, M. P. W. (n.d.). *Marjorie Phillips Wood, class of 1911 (B. Raab, Interviewer)*. [Audio file]. Pembroke Center Oral History Project. Brown University. www.brown.edu/initiatives/pembroke-oral-histories/interview/marjorie-phillips-wood-class-1911

Cameron, A. B., & Sherman, R. A. (n.d.). *Joint interview with Alita Dorothy Bosworth Cameron and Rowena Albro Sherman, class of 1914*. [Audio file]. Pembroke Center Oral History Project. Brown University. www.brown.edu/initiatives/pembroke-oral-histories/interview/rowena-albro-sherman-class-1914

Capelle, E. L. (1993). *Analyzing the "modern woman": Psychoanalytic debates about feminism, 1920–1950* [Unpublished doctoral dissertation, Columbia University].

Cushman, P. (1996). *Constructing the self, constructing America*. University of Michigan.

Dupont, J. (Ed.). (1988). *The clinical diary of Sándor Ferenczi* (M. Balint & N. Z. Jackson, Trans.). Harvard University Press.

Eliot, G. (1860). *Mill on the floss*. Harper & Brothers.

Everett, W. G. (1918). *Moral values: A study of the principles of conduct*. Henry Holt and Company.

Ferenczi, S. (1949). Notes and fragments (1930–1932). *International Journal of Psychoanalysis, 30*, 231–242.

Free Baptist Woman's Missionary Society. 1873–1921 (reprinted 1980). Unauthored Pamphlet, Providence, RI, Loose Leaf Manufacturing Company, 1922.

Free Will Baptists. (1834). *A treatise on the faith of the Freewill Baptists: With an appendix, containing a summary of their usages in church government.* https://archive.org/details/atreatiseonfait00goog/page/n27/mode/2up?q=we+claim+no+power+to+bind+the+consciences

Freud, S. (1952). *Sigmund Freud papers: Interviews and recollections, -1998; Set A, -1998; interviews and; Thompson, Clara, 1952.* [Manuscript/Mixed Material]. Retrieved from the Library of Congress, www.loc.gov/item/mss3999001575/.

From Brown Newsletter: Martha Mitchell's Encyclopedia Brunoniana. https://www.brown.edu/Administration/News_Bureau/Databases/Encyclopedia/search.php?serial=D0010.

Fromm, E. (1964). *Foreword* in Thompson (1964) *Interpersonal psychoanalysis: The selected papers of Clara M. Thompson* (Ed. Maurice Green, Foreword, Erich Fromm). Basic Books.

Goldin, C. (2006). The quiet revolution that transformed women's employment, education, and family. *American economic review*, 96(2), 1–21.

Green, M. R. (1964). Her life. *Interpersonal psychoanalysis: The selected papers of Clara M. Thompson* (Ed. Maurice Green, Foreword, Erich Fromm). Basic Books.

Hannah-Jones, N. (2019, August 18). Our founding ideals of liberty and equality were false when they were written. Black Americans fought to make them true. Without this struggle, America would have no democracy at all. *The New York Times Magazine*, 14(L).

Hawk, G. (1967). *Pembroke College in Brown University: The first seventy-five years 1891–1996.* Brown University Press.

Johnson, G. P. (1986, April 4). *Gladys Paine, class of 1913 (B. J. Anton, Interviewer).* [Audio file]. Pembroke Center Oral History Project. Brown University. www.brown.edu/initiatives/pembroke-oral-histories/interview/gladys-paine-class-1913

Layton, L. (2004). Dreams of America/American dreams. *Psychoanalytic Dialogues*, *14*(2), 233–254.

Marsden, G. M. (2006). *Fundamentalism and American Culture*. Oxford University Press.

Maslow, A. H. (1962). Some basic propositions of a growth and self-actualization psychology. In A. W. Combs & E. C. Kelley (Eds.), *Perceiving, behaving, becoming: A new focus for education* (pp. 34–49). Literary Licensing, LLC.

Mitchell, S., & Harris, A. (2004). What's American about American psychoanalysis. *Psychoanalytic Dialogues*, *14*(2), 165–191.

Parker, P. (2015). The historical role of women in higher education. *Administrative Issues Journal*, *5*(1), 3–14.

Perry, H. S. (1982). *Psychiatrist of America: The life of Harry Stack Sullivan.* Belknap Press.

Peterson, R. E. C. (n.d.). *Ruth Elizabeth Cooke, class of 1914*. [Audio file]. Pembroke Center Oral History Project. Brown University. www.brown.edu/initiatives/pembroke-oral-histories/interview/ruth-elizabeth-cooke-class-1914

Shapiro, S. (1993). Clara Thompson: Ferenczi's messenger with half a message. In L. Aron & A. Harris (Eds.), *The legacy of Sándor Ferenczi* (pp. 159–174). The Analytic Press.

Sprague, C. (2011, August 2). Explorer of inner space. *Provincetown Banner*, p. 37.

Thompson, C. (1915a, January 14). *Letters to Johns Hopkins University*. Adolf Meyer Collection 1890–1940; Series XV; Subseries XV/1; Sub-sub-series T. Alan Mason Chesney Medical Archives of the Johns Hopkins Medical Institutions, Baltimore MD.

Thompson, C. (1915b, September 28). *Letters to Johns Hopkins University*. Adolf Meyer Collection 1890–1940; Series XV; Subseries XV/1; Sub-sub-series T. Alan Mason Chesney Medical Archives of the Johns Hopkins Medical Institutions, Baltimore MD.

Thompson, C. (1947). Changing concepts of homosexuality in psychoanalysis. *Psychiatry, 10*(2), 183–189.

Thompson, C. (1958). Concepts of the self in interpersonal theory. *American Journal of Psychotherapy, 12*(1), 5–17.

Thompson, C. (1959a). An introduction to minor maladjustments. In S. Arieti (Ed.), *American handbook of psychiatry* (pp. 237–244). Basic Books.

Thompson, C. (1964a). Middle age. In M. R. Green (Ed.), *Interpersonal psychoanalysis: The selected papers of Clara M. Thompson* (pp. 335–343). Basic Books.

Thompson, C. (1964b). Childhood. In M. R. Green (Ed.), *Interpersonal psychoanalysis: The selected papers of Clara M. Thompson* (pp. 295–297). Basic Books.

Thompson, C. (1964c). Adolescence. In M. R. Green (Ed.), *Interpersonal psychoanalysis: The selected papers of Clara M. Thompson.* (pp. 298–304). Basic Books.

Chapter 3

On Becoming a Professional (1916–1920)

Clara Thompson must have been thrilled to write to Johns Hopkins Medical School and accept their invitation to join the class of 1920. She was an eager, interested learner.

> Dear Sir:
> Understanding that the number in each class of the Johns Hopkins Medical School is limed to ninety (90), I herewith acknowledge the acceptance of my application for admission and pledge myself to enter the first-year class in October 1916 . . . Signed, Clara M. Thompson, Address: 317 Jastram Street, Providence, R.I.[1]

That summer before starting school, she worked as a psychiatric aide at Danvers State Hospital in Massachusetts. Her exposure to psychiatry may have been the start of her career as a psychiatrist.

At Hopkins, she met the best and brightest psychiatrists, including her mentor, Adolf Meyer, who helped advance her career. At the end of her first year, she became a house medical officer. In 1923 she met Harry Stack Sullivan and introduced him to Adolf Meyer. She also met other women on a similar path in psychiatry who became her lifelong friends. For example, her friendship with Lucile Dooley opened new doors for her. She also became friends with Edith Jackson. (The details of her friendship with Jackson are discussed in Chapters 4 and 5.)

Johns Hopkins School of Medicine and Women

Thompson's acceptance to Johns Hopkins School of Medicine launched her life as a professional woman or, to use the expression of the time, a "modern woman." She wrote:

DOI: 10.4324/9781003261797-4

Not many years ago a woman's decision to follow a profession—medicine for example—was considered even by some analysts to be evidence of a masculinity complex. This rose from the belief that all work outside the home, especially if it called for the exercise of leadership, was masculine, and anyone attempting it therefore was trying to be a man.

Thompson (1942, p. 338)

Discrimination against women ran deep. She continued:

As early as 1850 a woman had "crashed" the medical profession. She was considered a freak and accused of immorality. Very slowly the number of women physicians increased. Still later, they entered the other professions and business.

(Thompson, 1941, p. 3)

The history of women at Johns Hopkins begins when Johns Hopkins Hospital hired faculty for a yet-to-be-built medical school. Enter the Friday Evening Club, five young women meeting twice a month in the 1870s. The women in their late teens and early twenties—Martha Carey Thomas, Mary Elizabeth Garrett, Elizabeth King, Mary Gwinn, and Julia Rodgers—shared an "interest in art, painting, literature and poetry." They were also feminists who "combined wealth and social position with a passion to improve the lot of women in America— and the know-how to do it. It was an advantage that four of the five had fathers on the board of trustees of Johns Hopkins" (p. 22). Mary Elizabeth Jarrett (2011) describes their connection to each other and to Hopkins:

The members of the Friday Evening Group all resolved never to marry. They felt that married women of that era were in bondage to their husbands, and they valued their freedom more than marriage. The one to break this vow was Mamie (Mary) Gwinn, but only after she and Carey Thomas had lived in a "Boston marriage" for some twenty-five years.

(p. 24)

These early feminists made an offer the medical school they could not refuse. They would raise the $500,000 needed to open the school and fund the cost for a building on the condition the school would open its doors to women. After much consternation, the school board agreed to the terms set forth by Mary Elizabeth Garrett. The Women's Fund Memorial Building was built in memory of the women (from the Friday Evening Group) who contributed to the higher education of women. They wished women to "enjoy all the advantages on the same terms as men" as well as "all prizes, dignities, or honors" given to male students. They wanted to commemorate the (October 28, 1890) date when the trustees of Johns Hopkins agreed to accept female students—by adding it to the school calendar. The medical school would exclusively be a graduate school and an integral part of the Johns Hopkins University. According to Garrett's conditions, the medical school would be a four-year-long training "leading to the Doctor of Medicine." Rigorous academic standards meant that students should have a background in the sciences and foreign languages of French and German. Students would have to pass medical courses to receive their degrees (Sander, 2008).

It was this group of feminists who altered medical education in the United States by insisting that 10% of the ninety medical school candidates each year be women. They also raised the criteria for admission for all students, male and female, to include a college education. In 1920, twenty-seven years later, Clara Thompson's graduating class had 13 women out of 90 students, slightly over 14%.

The Hopkins Medical School proved to be an exceptional educational environment for medical training. The Canadian physician William Osler had been recruited as physician-in-chief and the first Professor of Medicine of the University's planned School of Medicine. He established essential training procedures for advanced specialties and expanded the hospital's clinical services. Osler is famous for his insistence that the best student learning takes place not in the lecture hall but by seeing and talking to patients. He revolutionized the medical school curricula of the United States and Canada by adopting bedside clinical instruction as the primary method of medical teaching and learning. He established a medical residency program in the Johns Hopkins Hospital so that physicians would be supervised by trained doctors in their work with patients. Today's residency programs are a central component of post-graduate medical education, and for decades, his *Principles and Practice of Medicine* (1892) was the standard clinical medicine textbook.

Sisterhood in Medicine

By the time of Thompson's enrollment in 1916, Hopkins had achieved a stellar reputation. It set the standard for a more rigorous and scientific practice of medicine, fostered a "spirit of inquiry" and supported its graduates (Capelle, 1993, p. 170). Drawing closely on Capelle's (1993) discussion, we learn that, like Pembroke/Brown University—"the message to women students was mixed" (p. 171).

> Thanks to the stipulations of its feminist benefactors, whose contributions made its founding possible, the medical school had always admitted women, who remained for many years—in proportion to their numbers among the applicants—a constant ten percent of the ninety or so students in each class. The woman student would soon become aware, however, that there were few women in research or teaching positions at Hopkins or elsewhere, and that the majority of the internships and residencies that offered training for specialization were closed to women. (At Hopkins there were quotas on how many of these positions could be filled by women.)
>
> (p. 171)

Capelle speculates that women felt a particular affinity for the field of psychiatry because it was more welcoming and available to women than other specialty fields of medicine.

Thompson was one of an increasing number of women attracted to psychiatry. The Department of Psychiatry at Hopkins had a significant number of women in senior positions of responsibility on its faculty and in its clinics.

Like her classmates, Thompson was happy to embark on her chosen profession while simultaneously uneasy as to what shape her medical career might take. In a series of letters we hear from one of Thompson's friends, identified only by her initials JRC, an enthusiasm and a spirit of experimentation:

Clara dear,

I was much obliged to get your good letter. And I'm sorry that I can't accept your invitation . . . Today (Tues) I was in Boston where I saw the Board and made arrangements to borrow money; also I am taking up some work at Harvard medical in pharmacology which promises to be good with more interesting phases of the study of the effect of drugs on intestinal bacteria. I begin Thursday. I shall live at Hasseltine house (missionary home) at Newton Center. Will write more about this when I know more . . .

Dear Clara

I am studying Pharmacology. I don't know any yet but I intend to try my damndest to learn some . . . Mrs. White is an old lady who thinks God would show better judgment if he turned over the running of everything to her. However she isn't waiting for him to do so. If I had such folks to exhort me to become a Christian I should mortgage my clothes to obtain a partnership with the devil and commit myself to be sure of hell . . . Nevertheless, I am having a nice time and complying unprotestingly the cognomen of a "missionary doctor who is going to China" . . . That is where she decided I was going. But I don't care a straw. Last summer I should have been miserable here trying to get along conscientiously with this bigoted Christian tyrant, but I don't give a damn now. I feel a great deal of contempt for her waterproof ideas . . . I keep my own counsel . . . Friday morning I did an operation. Did you ever hear of anybody displaying such brazen nerve? Last Wednesday Mrs. White's laundress came and Mrs. White asked me to look at her arm which I found to be an infected gland in Rt. axilla and needing incision and drainage.

So I bought some iodine, some dichloride tablets, some gauze for dressing a 3-inch bandage, a tube of ethyl chloride and the dentist brought a scalpel. I sterilized everything in packages and Friday morning I went to the home of the victim where I did the operation . . . So far the patient survives. It was outlandishly high handed. But it was great fun. Supplies cost 2.05 but it was worth it for the fun. Love from JRC. August 15

Dear Clara

I suppose you are about to leave for home . . . I have attained some temporary decision . . . (a pleasant interruption by one of the girls bringing me three pieces of fudge, want to have a piece?)—I have a feeling of mixed recklessness and daring. Not caring what happens but ready to risk all. I'm staking everything on this year, or rather I am trying to throw everything into this next year, and "after us the deluge" is the sentiment. At the risk of your giving me another mark in favor of psy-choses . . . Mrs. Pamenter told me that I was one too much for her. It amuses me. But I have confirmed what was a sneaking suspicion that in the beginning, never give in or even compromise . . . Love from J.R.C.

These letters (housed in the Adolf Meyer Collection) express exhilaration and a resistance to the prevailing religiosity of the missionary house where this cohort of women boarded as they pursued their interests. Thompson's friend, JRC, grew to see through the hypocrisy of the religious zealots. Thompson most likely shared her views and she too rejected the religiosity of the Free Will Baptists.

Her Professional Life Faced Headwinds

The conflict between Thompson's strict early upbringing and her later wish for freedom from religious edicts, while most intense in college, also shadowed her years at Johns Hopkins. Green (1964) suggests that she became inwardly bitter and lonely, while outwardly appearing to enjoy the intellectual stimulation and familiar competitiveness of academic classes. The mixed messages regarding what women could hope to accomplish must have caused her concern.

When Thompson interned at the New York Infirmary for Women and Children (1921 22), she "wrote to her mentor at Hopkins [Adolf Meyer] that she was enjoying her work . . . "Things are going very well here and I am finding this year of general experience quite worthwhile" (quoted in Capelle, 1993, p. 172). Capelle (1993) points out that Thompson would have encountered Annie Sturgis Daniel, a physician and public health advocate for women and children. On seeing a connection between health and the social environment, Sturgis became a public reformer involved with local government who advocated for improving the lives of women and children as well as the status of women. Unfortunately, Sturgis held Victorian views about women and was a member of the old guard of early women doctors who demanded long hours of self-sacrifice. The work under Sturgis may have been of value but it also may have fueled Thompson's struggle with the prevailing cultural beliefs about women. In many ways, the theories of her profession were disloyal to her aspirations. Speaking directly to women in medicine, she wrote:

Women who studied medicine in the early years were on the whole those who had great personal problems about being women . . . there is a temptation to view all change as neurotic. This obviously is an extreme stand. Neurotic drives often find expression in the present-day activities of women, but this is no reason for dismissing as neurotic the whole social and economic revolution of woman along her particular path among the worldwide changes.

(Thompson, 1941, p. 8)

As to her struggle with self-esteem, she said:

Women . . . have had difficulty in freeing themselves from an idea which was a part of their life training. Thus, it has come about that even when a woman has become consciously convinced of her value she still has to contend with the unconscious effects of training, discrimination against her, and traumatic experiences which keep alive the attitude of inferiority.

(1942, p. 334)

The Influenza Epidemic of 1918

Thompson's years at medical school coincided with the influenza pandemic of 1918–1920. The virus ripped through the world with fatalities in adults in their 20s and 30s, Thompson's cohort. The soldiers at Camp Mead[2] outside of Baltimore reported the first cases of influenza. Baltimore newspapers focused first on the military cases at Fort Mead. Within days 1,900 soldiers were infected. The mayor of Baltimore, James Preston, and his health officials wrongly assured the residents of the city they were safe. The virus spread to other military bases and to Baltimore, where thousands of civilian contract laborers and their families became infected. Within a short time, the number of new cases overwhelmed the city hospitals. Residents were asked to donate sheets, blankets, and pillows for a makeshift hospital to help with the overflow. Quickly, it too was overwhelmed. Schools were closed, public gatherings were prohibited, churches and poolrooms were closed. Masks improved hygiene and social distancing was used to keep the virus at bay. Some families could not afford the expense of one or more funerals, and so the health department allowed burial without embalming. Crowded housing and unsanitary conditions placed many of Baltimore's newest immigrant population at greater risk. Some government officials were afraid that a closure of businesses would be worse than the epidemic itself. Racism prevailed. According to The University of Michigan Center for the History of Medicine, *The American Influenza Epidemic of 1918–1919: Baltimore, Maryland:*

> Except for Johns Hopkins Hospital and Bay View (for the city's poor and insane), the city's African Americans were admitted to Black-only hospitals. This color line affected not only the sick, but the deceased as well. By October, the city's African American cemetery, Mt. Auburn, was overwhelmed with caskets and not nearly enough graves. Few city employees were willing to dig graves for Blacks. When a call for volunteer gravediggers went unanswered, Mayor Preston appealed to the War Department for assistance. In response, 342 African American soldiers, along with a minister, were assigned the task, which they completed in a single day.

Masks were a major line of defense.[3] They were either mandated or required in cities across the country. The media back then discussed how to purchase, wear, and make masks with a clear focus on women. A gendered narrative promoted in hundreds of newspapers in the country showed an image of a Red Cross nurse wearing a mask. It suggested that the mask could be a fashion item able to conceal and hide facial flaws and enhance a woman's sexual appeal.

Thompson was fortunate to survive the epidemic, but it must have taken a psychological toll on her, and her cohort of young physicians. Back then, a similar attempt at denial and minimization of the dangerousness of contagion and infection was propagated by some government officials as in 2020. We do not know how Thompson weathered the trauma of that period either personally or as a professional.

A Positive Influence: Lucile Dooley

As mentioned before, during medical school, Thompson made important and lasting friendships with several women. Lucile Dooley[4] (class of 1922) became a life-long friend. Dooley (1884–1964) grew up in Kentucky and Tennessee. Her cousin George McMillian described her as a quiet person, who was "content" to teach (Burton, 1998, p. 51). This low-key description tells us little of the woman who was at the forefront of the development of psychoanalysis in America. Burton's (1998) biographical history of Dooley includes her cousin's notes. She describes the difficulty she had in obtaining accurate information about Dooley's life.

Dooley was one of seven children and her father's favorite. Like Thompson, she lacked a nurturing mother in her life. Her father was a major presence. She received top grades in school, drawing the attention of "older male supervisors and professors. In contrast, for many years, her female supervisors and teachers typically did not recognize her talents" (p. 56).

Following college she majored in psychology and attended Bible Teacher's Training School in New York City. Her supervisor was a psychologist named W.W. White. He encouraged her to attend Freud's lectures at Clark University in 1909. In 1911 she went as a missionary to Japan, where she became homesick and "had a nervous breakdown." She returned to Tennessee and enrolled in the University of Tennessee and obtained a master's degree in psychology. In the summer, she worked as an intern at L. Pierce Clarke's sanitarium in Stamford, CT, where she did "analytic work" under Clarke's supervision and became his analysand. In 1916, Dooley worked on a doctorate in psychology under G. Stanley Hall at Clark University. During her summers, she was employed as a therapist at St. Elizabeth's Hospital in Washington, D.C., where she impressed William Alanson White with her skills as an analyst and he urged her to go to medical school. She enrolled at Johns Hopkins and met Clara Thompson; the two became good friends. Dooley helped to recruit Clara Thompson and Anna Danneman Colomb as residents at St. Elizabeth's. Burton (1998) writes, "in Dooley's records and in my interviews with people who knew her, there was no mention of any romance in her life. Instead, she seemed married to her career" (p. 54).

Dooley, Thompson, and Colomb each attained significant prominence in the field. Anna Danneman Colomb founded the New Orleans Psychoanalytic Institute and served as its first Director. Dooley was president of the Washington Psychoanalytic Society. Her photograph is displayed along with all the former presidents of the Washington Psychoanalytic Society at the Society's headquarters (Burton, 1998).

Burton (1998) says that Dooley experienced severe and even suicidal depression. Following graduation from Hopkins in 1922, she remained in Washington and started a second analysis with Nolan Lewis. In 1931, she traveled to Vienna to spend a year as a candidate at the Vienna

Psychoanalytic Institute, where she consulted with Freud. He did not have time to see her so he referred her to Ruth Mack Brunswick. Dooley's life was entwined with other prominent psychoanalysts:

> Vienna was a woman's world for Lucile. Initially she lived alone in a pension in Vienna. When she became seriously ill with food poisoning, she asked her American colleague, Edith Jackson also a student at the Institute, for help. [Edith Jackson was also Clara Thompson's friend.] (Jackson had been analyzed by Dooley for a few years earlier in Washington D.C.
>
> (Burton, 1998, p. 66)

As Burton (1998) tells the story, "Edith arranged for Else Pappenheim's mother to nurse her back to health in the Pappenheim home" (p. 66). There she met and became intimate friends with Lotte Franzos who was married. After her husband's death, Franzos emigrated to Washington to live with Dooley. They remained together until Lotte died in 1954.

> Although Lotte and Lucile "never had a sexual relationship, they deeply loved each other . . . Lotte . . . took care of Lucile's personal and business needs . . . she would shop, cook, and houseclean for Lucile. She attended to all Lucile's correspondence and bookkeeping. Every morning and night she would brush out Lucile's long hair for her.
>
> (Burton, 1998, p. 68)

Following a classical line,[5] Burton maintains that through her relationship with Lotte, Dooley was able to "tap into deeper levels of creativity within herself." She suggests that "on a symbolic level" Dooley gave "her mother figure, Lotte, 'a baby' by way of the papers she conceived with Lotte's support" (Burton, 1998, p. 58).

Burton (1998) suggests (citing a personal communication from Pappenheim) that Dooley held "contemptuous feelings about Sullivan and his followers." But from Green (1964) we hear that Dooley was very taken with Thompson.

> Dr. Dooley, touched by [Thompson's] eagerness and intense intellectual curiosity, willingly shared her knowledge with Clara. She also

invited her to spend the following summer working at St. Elizabeth's Hospital in Washington, D.C. where she herself worked summers, and Clara enthusiastically accepted the offer to do so.

(p. 352)

Capelle (1993) also comments on Dooley's influence on Thompson:

Inspired by Lucile Dooley, Thompson went to Saint Elizabeth's Hospital for the summer clinical stint that was customary for Hopkins medical students between their third and fourth years. William Alanson White, an eclectic psychiatrist, encouraged his staff to experiment with various approaches to the treatment of mental illness. At Saint Elizabeth's, Thompson, like Dooley, worked under Edward J. Kempf, [who she later recalled as] "probably one of the first people to apply psychoanalysis through the treatment of psychotics in the United States."

(p. 178)

The circle of female friendships among these early pioneering psychoanalysts has yet to be fully explored.

Thompson Meets Thompson

During her third year at medical school, Clara Thompson met Joseph Chessman Thompson, a psychiatrist and American-born analyst who trained at the Washington-Baltimore Psychoanalytic Institute. They met when he was working at St. Elizabeth's Hospital. Although they shared the same surname, they were not related. Green (1964) describes him as a "kind man, sympathetic and compassionate" (p. 352). Joseph Thompson was an 1892 graduate of Columbia Medical School and had joined the Navy in 1897, reaching the rank of commander. He was a naval surgeon with wide interests who underwent psychoanalysis with Dr. Henry Grovens in 1923. He was also an associate of Abraham Arden Brill, Franz Alexander, and William Alanson White. It was he who saw Clara Thompson's unhappiness and encouraged her to get psychoanalytic help for herself by going into treatment with him.

Joseph Thompson had a depth of knowledge in a variety of fields, including Asian religion and zoology. He was known as "Snake" because of his interest in herpetology and was a founder of the San Diego Zoo.

Benveniste (2006) reports that Thompson gave "16,000 snakes to the Fleischacker Zoo in San Francisco" (p. 197). He was a recognized breeder of Siamese cats and was instrumental in developing the Burmese breed.

Raised in Japan by a missionary father, he shared with Clara Thompson the experience of religious restrictions in his youth. He could speak Japanese and read Sanskrit, and he was very interested in Buddhism, publishing on the subject under a Chinese version of his name, the pseudonym, Joe Tom Sun (Sun, 1924).

As a psychoanalyst, he held some unorthodox views. Publishing in naval medical journals, he compared Freud's early libido theory to the "procreation instinct" and "the steam generated in a boiler." This led him to posit ideas about psychological distress (Sun, 1924, pp. 319–327).

His views were quirky, ahead of his time, and unpopular. He felt lay analysts were equal to physicians in psychoanalysis. His support for lay analysts may have set the stage for Clara Thompson's long struggle to admit non-physicians into psychoanalytic training.

In 1924 at his suggestion, Clara Thompson began analytic treatment. Under Thompson's attention and influence, she may have experienced some relief from her internal struggles. Green (1964) reports that "her classmates, who had always known her as rather bitterly unhappy and alone, were impressed with the great rapport that she had with her analyst" (p. 353). Thompson's relationship with her analyst appeared to mitigate her loneliness and unhappiness. They were known to walk arm in arm around the campus at Hopkins and to dine together. The optics of their relationship led some, including Clara Thompson's advisor Adolf Meyer, to suspect them of having an affair, which Clara Thompson denied. To Meyer, their relationship did not pass an "appearance test."[6]

Residency Years (1922–1925)

Thompson began her three-year residency in psychiatry at Hopkins' Phipps Clinic in 1922. There she held the titles of Assistant Resident in Psychiatry and Instructor in Psychiatry. During her residency, she met some of the most innovative people in American psychiatry.

In the 1920s, Adolf Meyer was a dominant figure in American psychiatry.[7] He was Thompson's supervisor, but not a fan of psychoanalysis. He had advised her against becoming a psychoanalyst because he thought that would prevent her from securing a university position (Sprague, 2011).

As Thompson (2017)[8] summarized:

> Psychoanalysis was just beginning to be recognized outside of Europe and had caught the attention of many psychiatrists. Much of Freud's thinking was creeping into the orientation of psychiatrists in America. The importance of the experiences of early childhood in producing later difficulties was being stressed. Freud's concept of the unconscious, resistance, repression, and transference were beginning to be considered in observing patients. Meyer did not subscribe to Freud's idea of transference as a sexual attachment to the analyst. In fact, he hoped the whole problem could be avoided by a frequent change of therapist, thus discouraging too great attachment to any one person.
>
> (p. 488)

Fortunately, Thompson also worked under William Alanson White, the superintendent of St. Elizabeth's, and his associate Edward J. Kempf. Both men took to psychoanalysis early on. White encouraged all those working with him to use psychoanalytic concepts experimentally in working with psychiatric patients. Kempf had been doing this for years and had published two books on psychoanalytic work with patients (Green, 1964).

Adolf Meyer

The Swiss-born Adolf Meyer, an influential psychiatrist, first practiced neurology and taught at the University of Chicago. He was exposed to ideas of the late 19th-century Chicago functionalists, who stressed the importance of empirical, rational thought over an experimental, trial-and-error philosophy and the philosophy of William James. He was influenced by the ideas of John Dewey and James Angell, founders of the Chicago school of functional psychology. For a time, he was at the state hospital in Worcester, Massachusetts, publishing papers in neurology and psychiatry. He became the director of the Pathological Institute of the New York State Hospital system (also known as The Psychiatric Institute). Meyer was a professor of psychiatry at Cornell from 1904 to 1909 and then in 1913 became the founding director of the Henry Phipps Psychiatric Clinic at Johns Hopkins Medical School. He remained at Hopkins until 1941. He was president of the American Psychiatric Association from 1927 to 1928.

Meyer was strongly influenced by his wife, Mary Brooks Meyer, a social worker, who had recognized the important contributory role of social factors in psychiatric illness and treatment. Because of her advocacy, Meyer supported the incorporation of the innovative social service program at Johns Hopkins into the Henry Phipps Clinic and advocated for home visits. He initiated taking a complete social history of the patient, which proved to be a valuable component of the patient's integrated treatment plan. The result was a leap forward in psychiatry. Lamb (2015) summarizes:

> Meyer revised scientific medicine's traditional definition of clinical skill to serve what he called the "new psychiatry", a clinical discipline based on the principles of biological adaptation, and that shared social ideals with other 'new' progressive reform movements in the United States.

(p. 443)

Capelle (1993) recounts:

> Thompson first encountered Meyer when she took the required Introductory course in his department during her second year at medical school, and she went on to take elective courses in psychiatry during her last two years. After graduation, she served a year as a psychiatry intern at the Phipps Clinic, one of [the only women among thirty interns at Hopkins], and after completing her medical internship at the New York Infirmary the following year, she returned to Hopkins to become a psychiatric resident. She also served as an assistant dispensary psychiatrist, and in due time as an instructor on the faculty. In his letter of recommendation to the New York Infirmary, Meyer wrote that Thompson "had a very good standing in her class at graduation, and I have known her ever since her second-year course as a very good worker, conscientious and ambitious, and I greatly value her work at the present time."

(p. 176)

While rejecting many tenets of psychoanalysis, Meyer, as Thompson (2017) notes, encouraged those working under him to use Freud's methods. He did not "subscribe to Freud's idea of transference as a sexual attachment to the analyst" (p. 488). But he did agree with the importance of early childhood experiences and their influence on adult personality. As Waugaman (2014), noted, Meyer "had the innovative if quirky idea of trying to forestall the development of transference by frequently reassigning patients to new therapists" (p. 25).

Thompson's Relationship With Meyer

During the third year of her residency, Thompson became an instructor in psychiatry. Adolf Meyer, her supervisor, chose her to oversee his private patients while he was away. This was one of the highest honors one could receive as a psychiatric resident at Phipps. He initially saw her as conscientious and ambitious. His emphasis on open-mindedness must have appealed to her. Meyer was no fan of "the over-rigid New England conscience and the stern sense of duty and nothing but duty" (Capelle, 1998, p. 80) prevalent at that time. Thompson grew close to him and confided in him. His invocation to seek answers to life's questions in science must have fit with her Pembroke training to not take "ideas off the counter."

From Brennan (2015) we learn something more about Thompson and Meyer's relationship. He tells us that Meyer supported Thompson's interest in working with psychotic patients and that he "nursed" her through typhoid fever when she was "suicidal" (pp. 82-83).[9]

Was she suicidal? There is a spectrum of suicidality, and we don't have many details here. We know she was physically ill with typhoid fever and that could have colored the situation. At the time she was preparing her first paper on the topic of suicidal attempts in persons with schizophrenia. Brennan (2015) quotes a letter written by Thompson thirty years later (March 27, 1953, letter to Elsa Sprague Field), where she tells Sprague, "it's curious how a building [the Phipps Clinic] holds a memory. I think I can say the years of my greatest despair were spent in those walls" (p. 92). Thompson's unhappiness has been mentioned many times but now we understand that she was experiencing despair. Meyer noted in a letter (November 1, 1925) that Thompson "had a rather detached existence not making very close relations with other women at the clinic" (p. 92). By then, however, his evaluation of Thompson was likely influenced by her attachment to Joseph Thompson, who he strongly disliked, and by her interest in psychoanalysis rather than psychiatry. He could also have been jealous of her new closeness with her analyst. Writing about this period, Thompson notes:

> I had the privilege of psychoanalyzing a manic patient. The patient didn't learn anything, but at least I had my introduction to what was supposed to be psychoanalysis in those days . . . this was the beginning of a long sparring relationship with Adolf Meyer, because he did not want to discourage me but he didn't want quite to accept me either. So I was always being asked to compare his methods with Kempf's, and since I was just a green graduate, you can imagine that I had my difficulties. However, I spent four years in his [Meyer's] clinic.
>
> (Capelle, 1993, p. 178)

Going against Meyer's views was very difficult for her; he had been an important mentor to her and then he gradually turned against her. She officially resigned from the clinic on October 23, 1925, writing:

> I wish to hereby tender my resignation from the various positions I hold in the Phipps clinic—this resignation to take place at once. Sincerely, Clara M. Thompson.
>
> (Adolf Meyer Collection, 1890–1940)[10]

On October 31, 1925, Meyer responded:

> Your resignation is accepted . . . I cannot help feeling that, besides your own neglect of open discussion, a misleading influence kept you from a course of frank and direct inquiry and dealings. It may be the type and standard of psychoanalysis you have espoused, to venture on interpretations where it would be easy to get the facts directly.
>
> I do not ask for evidence of gratitude for what I have attempted to do at various times, although I should have appreciated some practical demonstration of responsibility. It was deplorable that you could disregard as you did the spirit with which you always dealt with. I regret especially that it does not become possible in this way to wipe out a record of actual and tacit misrepresentations and misjudgments that undermined your relations with the Clinic. A method of hasty interpretation which you tended to endorse has created much trouble for Dr. Harkin (who finally straightened it out) and has proven disastrous to

you using a wide range of opportunities to which I was willing to give my sincere support, although not an uncritical support. I appreciated your work, but deplored the influence of your associations.

Sincerely yours (Meyer Collection, 1890–1940)

Meyer's erratic personality may be another reason for the deterioration of Thompson's relationship with him. A letter from Lawrence Kubie to Ralph Crowley (Ralph Crowley's papers, March 1, 1971) sheds light on Meyer's personality:

It gradually became clear that Meyer fluctuated between warmly outgoing and communicative periods on the one hand to deeply angry, depressed, withdrawn and almost paranoid states on the other. These swings were long lasting, some of them lasting three and four years at a time. Therefore, the discrepancies between the accounts of what it was like to be a house officer in Phipps varied from black to white, depending upon the phase of the professor's neurosis through which he is passing.

Despite their differences, Thompson learned a great deal about the treatment of seriously mentally ill patients under Meyer's tutelage. Indicative of her character and attachment to him, she reached out to him a year after her dismissal inviting him to a meeting held at her apartment in Baltimore. Was she was trying to win him over to psychoanalysis when she wrote:

You are invited to attend a meeting for the organization of a Baltimore Psychoanalytical Society at my home on Thurs. Jan 21 at 8 p.m. Dr. Graven of St. Elizabeth's who has recently returned from study abroad will give a paper.

A reply is requested.

Clara M. Thompson. (Thompson, 1926)

Meyer declined.

Meyer's Revenge

Meyer maintained he appreciated Clara Thompson's work even as he pressured her to leave. According to Green (1964), Meyer repeatedly asked her to end her treatment with Snake Thompson, but she refused. He felt their walks and dinners together were a source of rumors around campus, giving the perception that they were having an affair. Meyer appears to have tried to destroy her career after that. On November 30, 1925, the year she resigned, he wrote a letter to Dr. Van der Chijs in Amsterdam, the Netherlands, denouncing her and turning away someone she referred to the Clinic.

My dear Dr. Van der Chijs:

I regret to say that Dr. Clara Thompson's connection with the Clinic had to be severed on account of an attitude that seemed to me incompatible with the interests of the Clinic. I doubt whether it would be right to encourage Miss van Laven to come here under the circumstances.

I find it exceedingly difficult to get the combination between psycho-analytic training and the type of make-up that limits itself to a critical sharing of experience without going over into vagarious or one-sided allegiances. I regret very much having to decline your request in this way, but I hope you will agree with me that under the conditions this is the wisest decision.

Believe me, With my best regards,

Very truly yours.

signed Adolf Meyer (Meyer (1921),
Correspondence 1890–1940)

The following year, on May 19, 1926, he wrote to a potential employer, Dr. Warfield T. Longcope:

My dear Dr. Longcope:

Dr. Clara Thompson resigned from the Clinic last October or November, and I allowed the resignation to pass because at the time I did not actually know that, in addition to matters which would have made continuation of service impossible, she had since June treated one of several patients of the Clinic for a fee of $100 a month at the offices of a clever but unsavory psychoanalyst, a Navy recruiting officer who was a U.S. spy in the Orient during the War. If any other facts were needed to settle the question of further connections with the Johns Hopkins Hospital,

I should let you have them. It was only by accident that I heard of her working in the Neurological Dispensary. Had her name come up before the Board, I could not have allowed it to pass, and I am sure you would have concurred with my suggestion that the application should be turned down.

I suppose Dr. Ford did not know the details of the situation when he took her in. But even so, I do not consider it a very thoughtful and even a very friendly step on his part. He must have known something of the situation and also how she neglected the neurological aspect of the cases to a remarkable extent. She is bright, but unduly free of some traits we would like to consider obligatory. I wanted to speak to Dr. Ford but was taken ill before I could reach him. I hope to be on deck again in a few days and shall try to see him then.

Believe me

Very truly yours (Meyer, A (1921),
Correspondence 1890–1940)

Longcope responded on May 20, 1926:

Thank you very much for sending me the facts concerning Dr. Clara Thompson, which I had not known previously. Her records naturally make it quite impossible for us to accept her in the Neurological Division of the Medical Dispensary and I will immediately speak to Dr. Ford about the matter.

Sincerely (Meyer (1921),
Correspondence 1890–1940)

Four years later, during her treatment with Ferenczi, Thompson tried again to reconcile with Meyer. In a letter to him, she described what she thought happened. Her attachment to him was similar to her attachment she had to her father. She received his support in her younger years but not as she grew older. Her parents too disapproved of her when she showed signs of having a mind of her own. Meyer was disapproving of her independence as well, and she was likewise resentful. In their correspondence, both sides are revealed.

November 12, 1929

Dear Dr. Meyer:

Four years is too long a period for a misunderstanding to exist without at least an attempt at understanding. I realize that it is largely my fault that no such attempt has been made and it is in order to correct that fault that I am writing this letter.

I do not of course know whether you desire to reestablish any contact with me and if you do not, of course, I know whether you may simply ignore this letter. For my part, it would be a xx action to me to explain to you the real facts of my mistakes in the situation and those which seemed to me to be yours and to give you a similar opportunity. Then I feel that even should we not wish to be friends, we can respect each other.

Should that wish be similar to yours I shall be glad to come over and talk with you sometime. It would be necessary to let me know about four days in advance so that I may arrange my appointments. Between 1.15 and 3.15 are the hours most satisfactory to me with the exception of next Tuesday.

Sincerely, Clara Thompson (Meyer (1921),
Correspondence 1890–1940)

A month later she wrote an additional hand-written letter.

December 7, 1929

Dear Dr. Meyer,

I was glad to receive your letter. I was surprised that you seem to have expected an answer to the one you wrote me four years ago. I have not the letter at hand so cannot quote exactly, but I remember quite distinctly one sentence to the effect that-it would be difficult even if I wished to re estab- lish relative of confidence with you and the clinic. It seems to me that such a sentence might discourage even a more aggressive person than myself. However since you now suggest that I might begin by answering that let- ter, and since some one must start the ball rolling if it is to roll I have no objection to your suggestion and will in general reply to what I can recall.

I suppose our real difficulty stripped of all the misunderstandings and tensions which developed later amounted to this—that you were hurt that I turned to psychoanalysis adopting a method of therapy not advocated or taught in the clinic, and that in addition I chose an analyst of whom you did not approve. I in turn was distressed at your disapproval but unwilling to alter my choice. The reasonable thing for one to have done under the circumstances would have been to have left the clinic as soon as possible—and that is what I would have done if it had not been for my attachment to you (transference) growing out of the fact that I had told my problems to you/verbally and, as in your method of treatment the transference is not analyzed. My attachment had continued to exist for several years. I was therefore confronted by two attachments and two individuals not friendly to each other, and I did not manage that situation very well. In my attempts to make a comfortable adjustment to you both I did you both an injustice. I suffered that the later situation between you and me was the direct result of the emotional tension which accumulated and made it untenable for us to talk frankly to each other—with the result that I possibly did unwise things and you were content to get indirect information about me rather than talking the matter of with me directly. In your letter you regretted the influence of our associates. Meaning I suppose my analyst. I am quite willing to grant that his judgment was not always the best, certainly partly due to the accumulated tension from which we were all suffering. I would criticize him as well as you and myself in the situation. I feel that if any one of the three of us had been able to view the matter non-emotionally many of the developments might have been prevented. This in general sums up my attitude toward the situation at the present time.

But to stop here would mean to leave certain things not clear. Therefore, I should like to mention specifically two or three things.

You said that I had caused Dr. Harkin trouble. This reference and our interview had with Dr. Werthemeier on the day before I left the clinic are not clear to me. Dr. Werthemeier in his conversation with me said that he had talked with Harkin and now he "knew all." I asked him what he meant and he would only reply that I knew perfectly well. The situation has always puzzled me and I would be grateful for an explanation. From what I know of Dr. Harkin's part history I can not believe that even if I did something unwise in my treatment of him, I could have been greatly responsible for his behaviors. But must <u>you and Dr. Werthemeier must have had something rather</u> definite in mind.

The next matter has to do with a <u>piece of gossip</u> which I heard two years after I left Phipps. It was reported to me that—that you said that you had asked me to resign because I was my analyst's mistress. I am not holding you accountable for a rumor. Of course, I suppose something was said by some member of your staff which formed the basis for it. But when I heard it I realized that it was a natural inference to have drawn from some of my behavior and that you probably believed it. A more sophisticated woman and one less secure in her innocence would have been more discreet. It happens that I have never been his mistress at any time. I do not know whether you can believe that and I do not know that it matters anyway, but since I am telling you facts that is one of them.

There is only one other thing that I want to mention that is your <u>having me removed from the neurology dispensary</u>. You may have thought you were justified in the step but it is very hard for me to take a natural attitude towards this. The problem was not my seeing Dr. Janeyhill invited me and made the arrangements. It seemed to me that either you feared I would do you some harm or it was purely an act of retaliation. The former idea seemed too ridiculous to entertain seriously considering our relative positions but when I think it was the latter it is very hard for me to keep an open minded objective attitude. Still, I have tried to do so in this letter and I hope you will reciprocate in the same spirit.

Sincerely, Clara Thompson (Meyer (1921),
Correspondence 1890–1940)

On December 10, 1929, Meyer responded, explaining his position:

Dear Dr. Thompson:

Your letter of December 7, 1929, brings out several points which undoubtedly deserve correction.

As to psychoanalysis, I was indeed distressed, not by the fact of your interesting yourself in it, but by your being unnecessarily blinded to important (in some case) facts not accessible to it. The choice of the analyst also had its share, and especially so because of the role you both, or at any rate the analyst, played in the Harken episode. The transference must have been ineffective on some essential points of allegiance—such as treating ward patients outside under conditions which the Hospital could not have tolerated. As to my being content to get indirect information about you, I am not aware that I acted in any essential point on hearsay. Some of the details are not absolutely fixed in my mind although I could probably look up such items as the threat of a suit against the Hospital or University on behalf of Dr. Harken by the man whom you allowed to come to a lecture with a stenographer. As to the "gossip"—I neither asked you to resign nor does it quite ring true that I should have given any such "reason" for what anyhow I did not do, or that I should deal in gossip on any occasion. I connect your resignation with a conversation you had with a member of the staff instead of your coming to me after that lecture.

The neurological dispensary decision was based on the fact that you had left without any explanation or attempt at mutual understanding and had not been appointed again by the Hospital, and I did not consider it appropriate that any one leaving one department in that manner should enter another department without a question being raised. It was not retaliation, but a combination of provocations of an official and not merely personal character.

These are to the best of my knowledge the facts and the motives of whatever I had a share in with regard to a frankly distressing experience, but not one governed by "emotional tension" at least on my part. My reaction to it was and is very much more objective than seems to have appeared to you. You can, I think, readily see that any getting together can only be on ground of a frank objectivity.

I no doubt have often said and felt that I have had a bad experience with a number of devotees of psychoanalysis. Why should I not look for a less seductive type of formulation? I have always had and have now a deeply rooted confidence in the supremacy of the wholesome tendencies in many patients too exclusively viewed for what is "wrong with them." There are more socializable ways of helping than "psychoanalysis" and I like to further them. In your own case you stopped on grounds of some superficial help you may have sought and obtained, and you prefer to work with conceptions handed out in a system too one-sidedly conceived and very effective at times, but only one of many reasonably effective methods.

I appreciate your letter as an attempt to eliminate emotionally tinged misconceptions. I trust that the objective facts I recall may put the entire issue on a more matter-of-fact ground.

Believe me

Very truly yours (Meyer (1921),
Correspondence 1890–1940)

This powerful exchange of letters ended their relationship. Despite her attempt to reconcile her relationship with Meyer, they never reached an agreement.

The Young Professional: 2025 Eutaw Place

As a young professional, Thompson settled into a Baltimore apartment at 2025 Eutaw Place and engaged a housekeeper, Ms. Lillie W. Fisher. (Their complicated relationship is discussed in *Clara M. Thompson's Professional Evolution and Legacy: An American Psychoanalyst (1933–1958)*.) She established a private practice and adopted a cat, making her home a cozy respite from her work. She supplemented her private practice income by teaching for two years at the Institute of Euthenics at Vassar College under Dr. Smiley Blanton.[11] Her teaching perhaps provided the extra funds she needed for her trip to Budapest.

Her home on Eutaw Place was in one of the most architecturally distinguished neighborhoods in Baltimore. Its buildings were turn-of-the-century row houses, mansions, and apartments of classically oriented design, the work of important local architects. They were home to some of the city's most important residents. She was surrounded by distinguished colleagues including Sullivan who had moved close by Joppa Road. That's when Sullivan met James Inscoe, who while underage (about 14 or 15) at the time later became Sullivan's life partner, Jimmie as he was known, and Harry would entertain Clara at their home weekly and, in turn, she would entertain them at her apartment (Perry, 1982).[12] Their lives were unconventional, she was a professional woman living alone, and Sullivan a distinguished psychiatrist living with a young man. Blechner (2005) describes

> People who admired Sullivan's thinking but were uncomfortable having a gay mentor, were happy to say that Jimmie Sullivan was just Harry Stack Sullivan's adopted son. But others knew there was much more to it, that Harry Stack Sullivan and Jimmie Sullivan were loving partners for more than twenty years.
>
> (p. 2)

Perry (1982) points out that some intellectuals and artists of the 1920s had a fear that marriage could destroy their lives and instead developed a different way of life. As an example, she mentions Gertrude Stein, and Alice B. Toklas, who set up alternative households. She avoids mentioning that these were gay couples.

> In that period, many young intellectuals with a sense of social responsibility, following the pattern already established by American artists, avoided marriage . . . Thus, one cannot view the early life experience of either Clara Thompson or Harry Stack Sullivan as a simple explanation for the pattern of living they adopted. They were indeed in tune with emergent attitudes about marriage as an institution in America, documented in part by Sinclair Lewis's novels.
>
> (Perry, 1982, p. 210)

Friendship With Harry Stack Sullivan

Clara Thompson met Harry Stack Sullivan in April 1923, when she was working at the Phipps Clinic. The meeting was unusual and awkward. Thompson was presenting her first professional paper, "Suicide and Psychotics." Later she described the meeting later:

> Apparently I looked like hell, and I was scared to death in addition, and Sullivan saw me and he thought, "My God, that woman is schizophrenic—I must know her!" . . . A few months later he got in touch with me and to his dismay I wasn't as schizophrenic as he thought.
>
> (Perry, 1982, p. 202)

Perry (1982) points out that Thompson's reference to being schizophrenic was both hyperbolic and a nod to Sullivan's saying that "all of us have full knowledge of the schizophrenic process, particularly in the adolescent year" (p. 202).

When they met, Thompson was 30 years old and Sullivan 31. They were both lonely people who were drawn to each other. While their early lives were different at least one outcome was similar, they rarely contacted their families of origin. Green (1964) says of Thompson: "Unlike the rest of us, who frequently spoke about our families, friends, and old times in school and hospital work, she seldom referred to the past" (p. 348). Perry found the same reticence in Sullivan.

Thompson and Sullivan were both gender non-conforming, she as an unmarried professional woman and he as a gay man. There were rumors about Thompson's sexuality, but the only hint of confirmation was in my interview with Zeborah Schachtel who confirmed Thompson was bi-sexual. They each must have felt society's disapprovals for gender non-conformity and gravitated toward each other as outsiders.

Part of being an outsider is dressing differently, claiming your own space. Green (1964) suggests Thompson neglected her appearance. It is clear she was not a fashionista; to me, the use of the word "neglect" sounds prejudice, or sexist. There are multiple references to Thompson's appearance that all bend toward "frumpy" or unfashionable. For example, Green recalls his first meeting with Thompson and describes her as, "a short, stout, plain woman" and Silverberg (1959) describes his first meeting similarly, though he adds more about her personality:

> A woman in her late thirties, who took no great pains about her appearance and made little effort to attract by such means. She was reserved, even shy, in her manner, but the sparkle in her eyes and the flashing beauty of her ready smile showed unmistakably a warm responsiveness.
>
> (p. 2)

In fact, Thompson wore what was then called "washfast" dresses.[13] These dresses were tailored and smooth fitting. They were described as having two stitched pleats in the front of the skirt and one stich pleat in the back. At the time, they could be purchased for between $3.77 and $27. The dresses needed little no special care and were worn for both dressy and casual occasions. Thompson, who was very practical, found them appealing.

Perry (1982) explains the closeness of Thompson and Sullivan's relationship in terms of Sullivan's developmental theory. She says that Sullivan found in Thompson "an eccentric girl who fits in with his peculiar restrictions and goes through the motions of the development of adolescent interests" (p. 204). This "combination leads to some of the most wonderfully eccentric relationships . . . these relationships can be very therapeutic" (p. 204). Perry surmises that Thompson and Sullivan found the "chumship" (p. 204) they needed to help them cross the line into the next phase of development.

Family Transitions

During the time Thompson was building her professional career, her younger brother Frank married Sarah Edith Borlase in 1929. Frank and Sarah, known as Peg, had two daughters, Sue (1932–2017) and Frances Dorothy (1934–2007). Both her nieces, like Thompson and her brother, attended Classical High School in Providence. Thompson would invite her brother's family to visit her in Provincetown during the summer months. She also enjoyed showing them around New York and taking in a play. Thompson's father died in 1930 at the age of 66. It was the year before she left for her longer stay in Budapest. It was after her father's death that she reengaged with her mother who lived another twenty years. Her mother died in 1952 at the age of 84, the same year Clara Thompson was interviewed for the Freud archives. Before her death, mother and daughter had reconciled enough to have visited and corresponded regularly.

Life in Baltimore

Thompson built a circle of friends in Baltimore. One of her friends was William V. Silverberg, who moved from Berlin to work at the Sheppard and Enoch Pratt Hospital in Towson, a suburb of Baltimore. He remembered living "practically around the corner from the spacious, but unpretentious walk-up apartment where Clara Thompson lived and practiced" (Silverberg, 1959, p. 3). Sullivan introduced Silverberg to Thompson, and they became close friends and colleagues. In his memorial tribute, Silverberg (1959) recalls:

> Clara's circle of friends in Baltimore in 1930–31 included, besides Sullivan and myself, Dr. Sam Wolman, his wife Adele, and Dr.

Marjorie Jarvis. Marjorie was a young and struggling psychiatrist. Sam Wolman was a prominent internist and was a good deal older than the rest of us, though his wife was more or less our contemporary. His interests, like those of his wife, were catholic and his information broad. An evening at Clara's or at the Wolman's generally consisted of excellent food, good company and lively talk about practically everything. We all liked music, and occasionally one of us would sing or play.

In about June of 1930, Sullivan took steps, at the instigation of A. A. Brill, to found the Washington-Baltimore Psychoanalytic Society. Clara accepted his invitation to join in this enterprise and was elected first President of the Society. During the winter of 1930–31, after Sullivan moved from Baltimore, a number of us working in psychoanalysis in Baltimore decided to meet every Sunday morning for informal discussion of difficult cases therapy. Clara was, of course, one of the group; some of the others were Lewis B. Hill, Eleanor B. Sanders, Marjorie Jarvis and Bernard S. Robbins, a resident at Sheppard. These discussions had such a uniformly and remarkably salutary effect on the therapy of her patients that we deduct this group in your club. I recall it as a thoroughly enjoyable and mutually instructive institution. In June 1931 Clara went to Budapest to continue her analysis with Ferenczi and it happened that we traveled on the same ship. I did not see her again until 1933 when she moved to New York. Sullivan had also meanwhile, moved to New York and I had returned and the three of us were much together during the ensuing years. We met regularly for dinner every Monday evening and called ourselves, following a whimsy of Sullivan's the zodiac club.

(Silverberg, WAW Newsletter, p. 3)

Silverberg also talked about the depth of their collegial relationships as he recalled:

During this period, Sullivan, Clara and I traveled to Washington or Baltimore once a month, sometimes twice a month to lecture, to conduct seminars or do individual supervision for the candidates of the Washington Baltimore-Psychoanalytic Institute; also, to attend meetings of the Washington-Baltimore Psychoanalytic Society . . . These jaunts were always great fun, apart from a more serious aspect, and we regretted having to give them up, in about 1936 . . . Clara and I were never again as close friends as we had been up to that time except the two years 1941 in 1943 what goes talk at the American Institute for Psychoanalysis we were nevertheless friendly and work closely together on such matters as the legal skirmishes with the American Psychoanalytic Association and the founding of the Academy of Psychoanalysis.

(Silverberg, p. 3)

In the same memorial newsletter of 1959, Janet MacKenzie Rioch recalled meeting Thompson at a meeting in Baltimore in 1934, the year after Ferenczi's death. She wrote:

Clara loved her work. Over the years, she brought to it a zest and energy and a sort of wide-eyed interest that was unfailing. The eager interest and incisive intellectual curiosity played an important part early in her professional life, for she then took certain steps that led to a great broadening [of?] her horizons.

(pp. 3–7)

During the fall to spring months of those years, as Silverberg describes it, Thompson was part of a group of Baltimore clinicians who met to discuss clinical concerns. Calling themselves the Miracle Club,[14] they were in effect a peer supervision group, a gathering of newly minted psychoanalysts striving for a more effective way to treat patients and to understand themselves.

In a footnote in her paper "The Role of the Analyst's Personality in Therapy," Thompson (1956) suggests:

I think that small group discussion of problems about patients can be profitably used by analysts all their lives. During the past few years, I have participated in a small seminar of graduates in which the emphasis is entirely on countertransference problems. It is a kind of miracle club, in which the participants swear the patient must have been listening in, because he reacts so often as predicted to the insight gained by the analyst.

(pp. 347–349)

Thompson's supervision group in Baltimore met each Sunday—until she left for Budapest in June 1931 to spend the next two years in psychoanalysis with Ferenczi.

Thompson's years in Baltimore were productive. She worked alongside many of the preeminent psychiatrists. She also was part of a growing group interested in psychoanalysis and a key participant as groups were organized into societies and training institutes in psychoanalysis. Yet despite all these professional associations and connections, something was missing from her life.

Finding Ferenczi

From 1926 to 1927, Sándor Ferenczi gave a series of lectures at the New School in New York City. Thompson with Sullivan heard Ferenczi's lecture, and she approached him about beginning an analysis. He did not have time to see her in New York but suggested she come to Budapest. Describing her thinking about that meeting, she said: "I went about, taught myself, I wasn't too unhappy, and then, honestly, I think it was February two years later, it went off like a bell in my head, and I thought I can go to him now" (see Chapter 1).

The revelation, "I can go to him now" has mostly eluded those telling the story of how she chose Ferenczi as her analyst. Green's (1964) account gives Sullivan prominence in the decision:

> Sullivan felt, like Meyer and White, that an unfortunate trend had set in there [in Europe] toward dogmatism and ritual. However, he had encountered one analyst, Sándor Ferenczi, who seemed to have avoided this trend. Ferenczi was coming to New York in the spring of 1927 to lecture at the New School for Social Research, and Sullivan advised Clara to see him at that time. She did this and, after talking with Ferenczi, arranged to undergo analysis with him.
>
> (p. 355)

Chapman (1976) gives a slightly different version. Thompson originally sought out Ferenczi herself when he lectured at the New School and invited her to come to Budapest for treatment. As we know, she followed through on that invitation in the summers of 1928–30. After that, Sullivan advised her to "go to Europe for extensive psychoanalytic training under Ferenczi" (p. 53).

Perry (1982) gives yet another version. Thompson told her,

> I would not have gone to Ferenczi [for my personal analysis] if Sullivan hadn't insisted that this was the only analyst in Europe he had any confidence in; and therefore, if I was going to go to Europe and get analyzed, I had just better go there. So I went.
>
> (p. 202)

Thompson sometimes minimizes the power of her own agency in actualizing her decision. She was drawn to what she heard from Ferenczi during those New School lectures.

This is when Thompson approached Ferenczi and asked him to see her for analysis while he was in New York. He replied that he had no time in the states, but he could see her in Budapest.

Her decision to begin psychoanalysis with Sándor Ferenczi not only changed the course of her career and personal life but also changed psychoanalysis.

Notes

1 This letter is from the Alan Mason Chesney Medical Archives of The Johns Hopkins Medical Institutions.
2 A digital encyclopedia produced by The University of Michigan Center for the History of Medicine, *The American Influenza Epidemic of 1918–1919: Baltimore Maryland*, (University of Michigan Center for the History of Medicine) notes that on September 24, 1918.
3 The nursing blog *Nursing Clio* (Brabble et al., 2020) points to how in 1918 masks were the major line of defense.
4 Dooley had obtained a doctorate in psychology under G. Stanley Hall at Clark University before medical school at Hopkins. She graduated a year after Thompson. Feeling unready or unable to return to Connecticut to begin clinical practice, she decided to remain in Washington in analysis. After two years, she still experienced severe and even suicidal depression. During her years in Washington, she worked at St. Elizabeth's Hospital, seeing psychotic male patients (see Lynn, 2003; Roazen, 1995).
5 Burton (1998) suggests that when Dooley was in treatment with Mack Brunswick, she developed an understanding of her desire for her mother, leading her to write: "It is the desire to hold the love object—usually mother but occasionally father that first leads to the exaltation of the penis in both sexes. The desire for the *person* . . . not for the organ is the dominant motive in the phallic phase in little girls" (1939, p. 192).

6 The appearance test did not hamper Freud and Ferenczi who frequently conducted "analysis" while walking in the countryside. But Thompson and Thompson's strolls around the campus did not receive the same acceptance.

7 Activity in the fledgling field of psychoanalysis was predominantly located in New York, under Abraham Arden Brill and "the only analyst west of New York" was thought to be Lionel Blitzsten of Chicago (Rubins, 1978, p. 168). (Blitzsten appears later in this story in his relationships with Karen Horney and with Harry Stack Sullivan (see Clara M. Thompson's *Professional Evolution and Legacy: An American Psychoanalyst (1933–1958)*).

8 This paper first appeared in *The Contributions of Harry Stack Sullivan* (P. Mullahy, Ed.), New York: Hermitage Press, 1952.

9 Brennan (2015) attributes this information to a letter to Elsa Sprague Field on March 27, 1953, held in "Thompson Papers, WAW." I was unable to find this letter at WAW.

10 Alan Mason Chesney Medical Archives, Johns Hopkins, Unit 1/3805.

11 She taught a course on Mental Hygiene (see Green, p. 354).

12 See discussion of Jimmie Inscoe in Drescher, J. (2017). Psychoanal. Persp., (14)(1):31–39 Smoke Gets in Your Eyes: Discussion of "When Harry Met Jimmie" Jack Drescher MD

13 Her friend, the psychoanalyst Zeborah Schachtel recalled these dresses in an interview, interview, January 12, 2016.

14 The members included Clara Thompson, Lewis B. Hill, Eleanora B. Saunders, Marjorie Jarvis, Bernard S. Robbins, and William V. Silverberg.

References

Benveniste, D. (2006). The early history of psychoanalysis in San Francisco. *Psychoanalysis and History*, *8*(2), 195–233.

Blechner, M. (2005). The Gay Harry Stack Sullivan: Interactions between his life, clinical work, and theory. *Contemporary Psychoanalysis*, *41*(1), 1–20.

Brabble, J., Ludwig, A., & Ewing, E. T. (2020, September 8). "All the world's a harem": Perceptions of masked women during the 1918–1919 flu pandemic. *Nursing Clio*. https://nursingclio.org/2020/09/08/all-the-worlds-a-harem-perceptions-of-masked-women-during-the-1918–1919-flu-pandemic/

Brennan, B. W. (2015). Out of the archive/Unto the couch: Clara Thompson's analysis with Ferenczi. In A. Harris & S. Kuchuck (Eds.), *The legacy of Sándor Ferenczi: From ghost to ancestor* (pp. 77–95). Routledge.

Burton, K. B. (1998). Lucile Dooley, MD. *Psychoanalytic Review*, *85*(1), 51–73.

Capelle, E. L. (1993). *Analyzing the "modern woman": Psychoanalytic debates about feminism, 1920–1950* [Unpublished doctoral dissertation, Columbia University].

Capelle, E. L. (1998). Clara Thompson as culturalist. *Psychoanalytic Review*, *85*(1), 75–93.

Chapman, A. H. (1976). *Harry Stack Sullivan: His life and his work*. Putnam Adult.

Dooley. (1939). The genesis of psychological sex differences. *Psychiatry*, 1: 181–195.

Green, M. R. (1964). Her life. In Green (Ed.), *Interpersonal psychoanalysis: The selected papers of Clara M. Thompson*. pp. 347–377 Basic Books.

Jarrett, W. H. (2011). Raising the bar: Mary Elizabeth Garrett, M. Carey Thomas, and The Johns Hopkins Medical School. *Baylor University Medical Center Proceedings, 24*(1), 21–26.

Lamb, S. (2015, July). Social skills: Adolf Meyer's revision of clinical skill for the new psychiatry of the twentieth century. *Medical History, 59*(3), 443–464.

Meyer, A. (1921). Letter to Clara Thompson. Adolf Meyer Collection 1890–1940; Series I; Unit I/3805, Folder 1,2,3. The Henry Phipps Psychiatric Clinic and Baltimore, MD. The Alan Mason Chesney Medical Archives of The Johns Hopkins Medical Institutions.

Meyer, A. (1925, November 1). *Notes on Clara Thompson*. Adolf Meyer Collection 1890–1940; Series I; Unit I/3805, Folder 1, unit 1/3882/1. The Henry Phipps Psychiatric Clinic and Baltimore, MD. The Alan Mason Chesney Medical Archives of The Johns Hopkins Medical Institutions.

Newsletter, William Alanson White Institute, W.A. White Psychoanalytic Society, 7(1) March, 1959.

Perry, H. S. (1982). *Psychiatrist of America: The life of Harry Stack Sullivan*. Belknap Press.

Rioch, J. M. (1959). Clara Thompson: Her professional life and work. *The Newsletter of the White Institute, 7*(1).

Rubins, J. L. (1978). *Karen Horney: Gentle rebel of psychoanalysis*. The Dial Press.

Sander, K. W. (2008). *Mary Elizabeth Garrett: Society and philanthropy in the gilded age*. Johns Hopkins University Press.

Silverberg, W. V. (1959). Clara Thompson memorial. *The Newsletter of the White Institute, 7*(1).

Sprague, C. (2011, August 2). Explorer of inner space. *Provincetown Banner*, p. 38.

Sun, J. T. (1924). Psychology in primitive Buddhism. *Psychoanalytic Review, 11*(1), 39–47.

Thompson, J. C. (1924). Tropical neurasthenia: A deprivation psychoneurosis. *Military Surgeon, 54*, 319–327.

Thompson, C. (1926, January 11). Letter to Adolf Meyer. Adolf Meyer Collection 1890–1940; Series I, Unit I/3805, Folder 1. The Henry Phipps Psychiatric Clinic and Baltimore, MD. Alan Mason Chesney Medical Archives of the Johns Hopkins Medical Institutions, Baltimore MD.

Thompson, C. (1941). The role of women in this culture. *Psychiatry, 4*(1), 1–8.

Thompson, C. (1942). Cultural pressures in the psychology of women. *Psychiatry, 5*(3), 331–339.

Thompson, C. (1956). The role of the analyst's personality in therapy. *American Journal of Psychotherapy*, *10*, 347–359.

Thompson, C. (2017) The history of the William Alanson White Institute. Contemporary Psychoanalysis, 53(1), 7–28. This paper was first given in 1952 for the Society.

University of Michigan Center for the History of Medicine. (n.d.). *City essays: Baltimore, Maryland*. The American Influenza Epidemic of 1918–1919: A Digital Encyclopedia. Influenza Encyclopedia. Michigan Publishing, University of Michigan Library. www.influenzaarchive.org/

Waugaman, R. M. (2014). Commentary on "transference as a therapeutic instrument": Remembering Sullivan's psychoanalyst. *Psychiatry*, *77*(1), 25–29.

William Alanson White Institute, W. A. White Psychoanalytic Society, 7(1) March, 1959.

Chapter 4

On Clara Thompson and *The Clinical Diary* of Sándor Ferenczi

Clara Thompson and Sándor Ferenczi were both psychoanalytic mavericks. In 1928, nearly two years to the day Ferenczi suggested Clara Thompson come to Budapest for psychoanalytic treatment, she thought, "I can go to him now." She hadn't given it much consideration since their initial meeting, but she had saved the requisite funds to finance her trip. "Why not go?" she asked herself. She prepared to be away for the summer and boldly set sail aboard the steamship Belgenland for the five-day journey. The German ship boasted a large veranda cafe, an elegant smoking room, a gym, children's playroom, an attractive lounge, and a library[1] suggesting that her trans-Atlantic crossing was quite comfortable.

Her arrival in Budapest marked the start of an extended period of self-discovery that includes the summers of 1928 (for two months), 1929 (for two months), 1930 (three months), and two full years from 1931 to 1933.

Thompson's Choice of Ferenczi as Her Analyst

Why did Thompson choose Sándor Ferenczi? What was she looking for in an analyst? What outcome did she expect? Perhaps, she would say her analysis with Ferenczi began when she heard him lecture at The New School for Social Research on *"Selected chapters in the theory and practice of psychoanalysis."* Or perhaps, even before then, when she heard her colleagues, particularly Sullivan, speak positively about him. It might have begun when she read one of Ferenczi's publications. In her essay, *"Notes on the Psychoanalytic Significance of the Choice of Analyst"* (Thompson, 1938), she says, "every psychoanalysis has a beginning, and patients often exercise what is called choice in selecting the person with whom they will

DOI: 10.4324/9781003261797-5

undertake the work" (p. 205). She said an analyst is generally chosen in one of several ways:

> (a) either on the advice of or through the indirect influence of another person; or (b) through some personal knowledge of or contact with a given analyst or group of analysts. When the advice comes from a third person, the individual influencing the choice may do so in a professional or friendly capacity . . . He may take this person's advice because he has confidence in his judgment, or for more complicated emotional reasons, such as fear, competitiveness, hostility, identification, love, etc . . . when an outside person does not influence the prospective patient, the choice may be made through reading an article, hearing a lecture, or by personal contact with the analyst before or at the first interview.
>
> (p. 207)

Thompson believed that choosing an analyst was complicated by both the personality of the analyst and the patient. This may seem obvious to us now but in 1938 these ideas were groundbreaking. She underscores an important quality in the choice of an analyst that often eludes discussion:

> the patient in quest of an analyst has his preferences . . . the analyst plays a part in the patient's choice, and that is the analyst's interest in him, the feeling of empathy . . . part of this interest or lack of interest may be imagined by the patient, but we do know that not all patients interest us equally, and that, by various devices, subtle and overt, those who especially interest us come most frequently to find their way into our practices. In short, some sort of natural selection takes place, and both analyst and analysand have a part in bringing it about.
>
> (1938, p. 207)

Thompson understood that what all patients seek in an analyst is:

> the person with whom they feel most capable of having an intense emotional relationship; that is, they seek the personality which most nearly corresponds to personalities with whom they tend to have attachment.
>
> (p. 208)

In her 1952 interview with Kurt Eissler, she said, "You see, my mother was the harsh one in my family. My father was very like Ferenczi."

Sándor Ferenczi and Sigmund Freud

Born in 1873 in Austria-Hungary, Ferenczi received his medical degree in Vienna in 1894 when he was only twenty-one. He served as an army physician specializing in neurology and neuropathology and was skillful in hypnosis before meeting Freud in 1908 (Rachman, 1997). Ferenczi was one of the six psychoanalysts Freud chose to advance the cause of psychoanalysis. He was "dearly loved" by Freud (Roazen, 1975, p. 10). As a rising star in psychoanalysis, Ferenczi became Freud's constant companion and was destined to be Freud's successor. He introduced the notion of empathy into psychoanalysis, for which he received Freud's full approval (Rachman, 1997).

Ferenczi was known as the "go to" therapist for difficult cases. His therapeutic approach took him beyond empathy to more active methods than traditional "on the couch" psychoanalysis (Perry, 1982). For Ferenczi, action fostered the development of theory rather than the other way around. He came to understand that therapy required an active role by the therapist in a give-and-take dialogue with the patient. Coupled with his understanding of trauma, an innovative treatment was developed that was a departure from Freud's therapeutic model. Thompson (1955) recounts that during the years she was in treatment with Ferenczi, he was working on his new techniques, "which were then known as 'relaxation' therapy . . . They were years of great stress and conflict for him" (p. 3), she adds, due to his departure from Freud's work.

Ten years after Ferenczi's death, Thompson (1943) paid tribute to him:

> I believe that Ferenczi pointed out things in need of emphasis in the analytic world. He was the only person in Europe at the time who saw some of them and had the courage to state them.
>
> (p. 64)

In her 1934 memorial essay, she reveals the depth of her feelings.

> In May 1933, there died in Budapest the greatest of Freud's pupils, Sándor Ferenczi, a man, great not only because of his remarkable intellect, imagination, and unquenchable scientific curiosity, but

also because of his profound simplicity, humility, and gentle human kindliness.

(Thompson, 1988, p. 182)

She believed,

> Ferenczi was impeded in developing his own thinking by the nature of his attachment to Freud—an attachment compounded of admiration, dependence, fear of disapproval, and veiled rebellion.
>
> Only his pupils, in private conversations, obtained an uncensored glimpse of Ferenczi's own thinking. This thinking deviated quite radically from that outlined in most of his published works. Then was he able to express his lack of enthusiasm for many of the Freudian concepts. He found them too theoretical, too difficult to apply, too unfriendly to the patient. He did not clearly see that he was questioning the validity of the instinct theory; he saw his disagreements with Freud rather in terms of practical applicability to the patient. For years, however, he was unable to speak of this publicly. He remained a secret rebel who could not quite allow himself to know of his rebellion.
>
> The need for approval, the need to be accepted by "the strong one," were therefore serious hindrances to Ferenczi's thinking. One feels that he betrayed some of his best ideas by attempts to avoid offending Freud. This resulted in unevenness and even some degree of insincerity in his writing.

She added,

> I have presented this summary of Ferenczi's relation to Freud in order to explain why so much of what was his original contribution to psychoanalysis was either never published at all or published in such a censored form that it must be difficult for those who did not personally work with him to understand.

(p. 186)

Thompson held both Freud and Ferenczi accountable for Ferenczi's inhibitions. Ferenczi was dedicated to helping people and to finding ways to alleviate human suffering. In his therapeutic efforts, he experimented with different approaches as he tried to discover what worked best. As he experimented—with Elizabeth Severn, then Clara Thompson, and his other patients, his methods diverged further from those practiced by Freud. During this period, he abandoned the role of the cool, detached classical analyst and embraced a relaxed, more human connection. He was passionate about discovering how to "cure" people of their psychological problems and hoped to reduce the length of time that standard treatment required. He valued subjective experience and focused on his own thoughts (countertransference), as well as those of his patients.

In his innovative work with patients, most notably Elizabeth Severn, he experimented with what they called a mutual analysis. During that period of work Ferenczi recalled that he had been sexually abused as a child by "a housemaid":

> [An] image of a corpse, whose abdomen I was opening up, presumably in the dissecting room; linked to this the mad fantasy that I was being pressed into this wound in the corpse. Interpretation: the after-effect of passionate scenes, which presumably did take place, in the course of which a housemaid probably allowed me to play with her breasts, but then pressed my head between her legs, so that I became frightened and felt I was suffocating.
>
> (Dupont, 1988, p. 61)

His recollections of sexual abuse during his mutual analysis with Severn may have played a role in his development of a theory of childhood sexual trauma, a theory that ultimately separated him from Freud.[2]

Freud initially believed that the traumas reported by his "hysterical" patients were true, but he later abandoned that belief, concluding that the fantasy of abuse was more frequent than the trauma itself. Rachman (2021) argues that Freud sacrificed understanding trauma by focusing instead on his oedipal theory of development. Ferenczi was the first to return to the idea that the root of most "neuroses" or psychological disorders begins with real trauma. His seminal *"Confusion of Tongues between the Adults and Child"* (1949a), a landmark paper in psychoanalysis, confirmed not only the reality of sexual abuse but its resulting sequelae.

Freud believed that Ferenczi strayed too far from his (Freud's) theories. As a result, for many years Ferenczi's contributions were sequestered and silenced. Ernest Jones (1957) collaborated in discrediting

Ferenczi by falsely claiming he had become psychotic (see Bonomi, 1999).[3] Before being marginalized, Ferenczi successfully managed to extend interest in psychoanalysis beyond Austria and Germany into Eastern Europe, where he was a founder of Hungarian psychoanalysis (Rachman, 1997).

Ferenczi's Technical Innovations

By the time Thompson arrived in Budapest in 1928, Ferenczi was already practicing what he called his "relaxation method" (Thompson, 1950a). As Thompson describes it, "Ferenczi developed his thinking in two phases— first a phase of active technique and later a phase of permissive technique, which he called "relaxation" therapy" (p. 182). He was acting on the assumption that what made people "neurotic" was that "they had never been accepted or loved as children." What they needed was the experience of love and acceptance.

She provides some descriptions of what this new phase entailed:

> The giving of five or ten minutes extra and in extreme cases even longer at times when a reaction has been extremely powerful and prostrating is an example, Another situation is seen in the case of a patient who was always very punctual. Her first lateness, due unmistakably to resistance, was accompanied by great anxiety and fear of disapproval. In order to express understanding of her true state of mind, the lost time was given her at the end of the hour as a present with an explanation of the meaning of the gift.
>
> (Thompson, 1964, p. 67)

Thompson admired Ferenczi's persistence and his willingness to be helpful. She felt that he was

> "Possessed of a genuine sympathy for all human suffering, he approached each new case with an enthusiastic belief in his ability to help and in the worthwhileness of the patient. His efforts were tireless and his patience inexhaustible. He was never willing to admit that some mental diseases were incurable, but always said, "Perhaps it is simply that we have not yet discovered the right method."
>
> (Thompson, 1988, p. 182)

Natural Expression in a Favorable Atmosphere

In her essay on "Ferenczi's Relaxation Method," Thompson (1964) discusses a patient who may be a disguised version of herself as a young girl:

> The first case is that of a woman who had grown up in an intolerant small-town community where childhood sexual activities with boys in her neighborhood brought her open disgrace and ostracism. At the time of the analysis, it was apparent that she wished to make her body unattractive and avoided, to an extreme degree, all physical contact. A time came in the analysis when not only did it seem important to talk of whether her body was repulsive to the analyst, but to test it. To this end she was encouraged to try a natural expression of her feelings. It seemed necessary for her to kiss the analyst not only once but many times and to receive from her not simply passivity but an evidence of warm friendliness and a caress in return before she could even become conscious of the degree of degradation she had felt.
>
> (pp. 67–68)

This vignette (with a change of the analyst's gender) may shed some light on an important component of Thompson's treatment with Ferenczi, discussed below.

Discovering the most helpful method became Ferenczi's passion. He had turned down the presidency of the International Psychoanalytic Association, a position that Freud encouraged him to assume in order to focus intensively on his clinical work. This decision was discussed by Freud and Ferenczi over a period of months, as Brabant (1993) confirms. At the same time, Ferenczi pressed Freud to continue his analytic work with him. Ferenczi was always wanting more analysis. However, a tension evolved between the two men that eventually led to a disruption in their relationship.

The *Clinical Diary*: A Look Before a Leap

A close examination of Ferenczi's *Clinical Diary*[4] offers an opportunity to hear Thompson's voice as the patient Dm., Ferenczi's reflections about Dm., and his views about psychoanalytic work.

Thompson (1955) states that Ferenczi's method of working on his ideas included "his students" thoughts and associations. She describes how Ferenczi kept his diary:

> He always had a wad of papers. Often during an analytic hour, a patient would say something, which either contributed new data about some thought on which he was working or clarified some issue. Out would come the pieces of paper and a note was made on the piece already containing thoughts on the subject.
>
> (p. 3)

In order to protect the privacy of his patients, Ferenczi used initials to disguise their identities.[5] However, Clara Thompson was mentioned by name (Dupont, 1988, viii) and also identified as Dm.[6]

Clara Thompson as Dm.: The Reliability of the Entries

With so much importance placed on the entries in the *Clinical Diary*, it is not unreasonable to question their reliability. Together with Arnold Rachman, I explored this matter in a letter to Judith Dupont on April 15, 2019.[7] Her response, dated April 16, 2019, sheds some necessary light on these entries. She writes:

> It seems obvious for me that the passage you quote concerns Severn rather then (sic) Thompson. The allusion to mutual analysis also seems to be in this direction. I consider this as a way of mixing clinical stories in the intention to make the identification of people concerned less easy. It seams (sic) that Ferenczi wanted his Diary to be published at some time, and for that reason he did not give the names of the patients but called them just by letters.
>
> As all this became not only a clinical study but also history, we wanted to know who is Dm., or RN, but it was not intended by Ferenczi to be revealed.
>
> That is all I could tell you about this "confusion" or maybe rather intentional mixing of the two stories.
>
> Sincerely yours,
>
> Judith Dupont

On April 17, 2019, she later added:

> What I can say about Ferenczi's intentions is pure hypothesis. It could be a possible explanation of the facts. As the Diary was written at the same time as he did the clinical work with the two women, it could only be a voluntary mixing. But I cannot guarantee the exactness of my explanation.

The Patient Thompson Emerges

A word of warning. There is much to unpack in the diary notations. They are challenging because they are thoughts and fragments not written in a linear fashion yet they are worth the effort to understand. References to Thompson begin on the first page of the *Clinical Diary*, where Ferenczi refers to "Groddeck-Thompson" by their given names.[8] Then, patient Dm. makes her appearance as the "lady" who Ferenczi allowed to "occasionally" kiss him. The patient "casually in the company of other patients, who were undergoing analysis elsewhere" then said, "I am allowed to kiss Papa Ferenczi, as often as I like." Next it is disclosed that, "As a child, Dm. had been grossly abused sexually by her father, who was out of control" (Dupont, 1988, p. 2-3). Dupont writes,

> an incident that came to Freud's notice via Clara Thompson, the patient in question, and which caused Freud to write the well-known letter of 13 December 1931. This letter has been often quoted since its publication . . . In it Freud reproaches Ferenczi for what he calls his "technique of kissing" and ironically points out some of the regrettable consequences that might result from its spread and its further development in the psychoanalytic world.
>
> (Dupont, 1988, p. 3)

These assertions have led to many assumptions and criticisms of Thompson, including that she was "at least indirectly, therefore, responsible not only for exacerbating the conflict between Ferenczi and Freud but also for much of the damage to Ferenczi's posthumous reputation" (Rudnytsky, 2015, p. 136). Rudnytsky also suggests that this "kissing episode" led some analysts to dismiss Ferenczi's work "as not psychoanalysis." On the positive side, he noted that Clara Thompson left a "lasting mark on subsequent generations of interpersonal analysts" (p. 140).

The Explosion

Thompson and Edith Jackson created a crisis when Thompson told her friend she could kiss Ferenczi anytime she wanted. Her friend Edith Jackson was in treatment with Freud. Jackson reported what Thompson told her back to Freud in much the same way that she brought back other information to him about his patients and his social circle. Comparing notes on what transpires in analysis is not uncommon in analytic institutes, where candidates exchange information often with the intention of expanding their understanding of clinical treatment. Of course, there is also plenty of gossip. Justifying her right to tell Jackson, Thompson said she believed Ferenczi needed to stand up to Freud and to speak openly about "what we do."[9]

Thompson in explaining Ferenczi's innovative "relaxation method," said it was as if Ferenczi was saying,

> I am interested in you not only as an adult patient, but I am interested in and have sympathy for the child part of you also. In the childish attachment you have formed for me, I will continue to be your interested friend.
> (Thompson, 1964, p. 67)

Ferenczi was encouraging the "reliving" of childhood experiences in what Thompson referred to as a "play technique" (p. 67). She was also invested in Ferenczi standing up to Freud and defending his clinical innovations. One wonders if she had also wanted her father to stand up to her abusive mother since she said she saw Ferenczi as being like her father and Freud like her mother.

This raises a set of questions: Did Thompson understand that Ferenczi was creating an empathic atmosphere to allow her to freely express her affectionate feelings when he permitted her to kiss him? Did Ferenczi, by not asking her to analyze her feelings or behavior, fail to make any (sexually) abusive behavior knowable? Was either Thompson or Ferenczi aware of a potential erotic transference and countertransference in allowing her to kiss the analyst? Thompson addressed some of the possible complications in her essay, *Ferenczi's Relaxation Method* (Thompson, 1964).

Thompson's childhood poem (see Chapter 2) may reveal something more about the evolution of the kiss. In Thompson's poem, she depicts a young girl shamed for expressing her affection. This poem sheds light on Thompson's need to be able to express her affection without being humiliated. Ferenczi's empathic response to her need was important. In that way, the kissing episode was in part a reparative experience.

Ferenczi did not initiate kissing Thompson. He allowed it as part of his relaxation method, fostering an open, accepting, empathic stance that allowed the spontaneous expression of all thoughts, feelings, and behaviors in the analytic situation with the intention of being without judgment, criticism, or need to interpret. He saw the passive, nonreacting, aloof analyst as repeating childhood trauma. "If the patient is ill because he had not been loved, the cold, passive analyst only continues the situation to which he is already accustomed; whereas an atmosphere of liking and acceptance would furnish a new experience and, in that setting, the patient could dare to face his unhappiness" (Thompson, 1988). Further, an analytic pose of infallibility repeats all too well the childhood situation when mother is always right, although the child often has good evidence that she is wrong. To Ferenczi, repeating this experience in the analysis only maintained the neurotic status quo. The patient's defenses were originally developed to cope with the insincerity of the parent and would continue with the insincerity of the analyst.

> With this in mind, Ferenczi set out to develop a therapeutic situation in which the patient might receive the acceptance and sincerity he had needed most in his childhood. Another point was also stressed. Since analysis was becoming too intellectualized, Ferenczi sought ways to encourage more emotional reliving, believing that only by the emotional reliving could the patient be cured.
>
> (p. 190)

Kissing Ferenczi

During her analysis, Ferenczi suggested to Thompson that she find a way to express her affection—she did, she kissed him. He graciously accepted her kisses. Despite the problems it caused him, her spontaneous expression of affection had a positive effect on her treatment. She reported in the Eissler interview that she found the whole treatment nearly 100% positive (Thompson, 1952). Before her analysis, she explains, she was detached and schizoid; after the analysis she was able to develop relationships with people though she felt she still had some difficulty with intimacy. Thompson tells a story about Ferenczi's special intuitive abilities that she thinks could help us understand how he worked. She says,

> During the war a soldier who was a personal acquaintance was being disciplined for some serious misdemeanor under the strain of

the disgrace the man developed an acute mental illness in which he became very slovenly neglecting all care of his body. On hearing of this, Ferenczi hastened to the man and completely disregarding his appearance embraced him and genuine concern intuitively without a word from the man he had seen his need of being reassured that a friend could like him no matter how great his disgrace the man's recovery began in that hour.

(Thompson, 1964, p. 66)

Presumably, drawing on his intuitive sensibility, Ferenczi felt Thompson needed to be encouraged to show her spontaneous affection—to trust that it would be <u>accepted</u> in the way that the soldier she described needed to feel accepted. He was correct. Her confidence was restored.

Thompson (1944) explained that Ferenczi believed "a person became ill because of what had happened to him."

(H)e claimed that he was revising Freud's early idea of infantile sexual trauma. Actually, however, Ferenczi's concept was more broad than Freud's earlier one. Not only did he consider early sexual experiences as significant in producing traumata, but he viewed many attitudes of parents toward their children as traumatic. Expressing the feeling that children especially suffered as a result of the insincerity of parents, he said, "Children know the truth before they learn the meaning of words. After they learn the meaning of words, they become confused.

(p. 247)[10]

Thompson's kissing Ferenczi has been referred to by Brennan (2015) as "a mutual enactment" where "Thompson replicated the dynamics of childhood boundary crossings and in particular, her own confusion between childhood tenderness and adult passion" (p. 84). Brennan suggests further that "Ferenczi was enacting his own desire to be the loving mother he never had" (p. 84). Sue Shapiro (1993) reading the Clinical Diary found two of her interests coincided, first, her interest in Clara Thompson and second, her work with survivors of sexual abuse. She concludes that Thompson became "a messenger with only half a message." (p. 167) She wished that her "psychoanalytic grandmother had brought Ferenczi's ideas about sexual trauma into her clinical work" (p. 159).

Freud, Ferenczi, and Thompson

This "kissing" episode preoccupies the psychoanalytic community generating assumptions about Clara Thompson's personality and behavior. First noted in the January 7, 1932, diary entry Ferenczi faults himself for adhering to a rigid protocol with previous patients. He acknowledges that a relaxed method, while helpful, can lead to "bad experiences," and he gives examples. He writes about patient Dm. (Thompson):

> See the case of Dm. a lady who, "complying" with my passivity, had allowed herself to take more and more liberties, and occasionally even kissed me. Since this behavior met with no resistance, since it was treated as something permissible in analysis and at most commented on theoretically, she remarked quite casually in the company of other patients, who were undergoing analysis elsewhere: I am allowed to kiss Papa Ferenczi, as often as I like. I first reacted to the unpleasantness that ensued with the complete impassivity with which I was conducting this analysis. But then the patient began to make herself ridiculous, ostentatiously as it were, in her sexual conduct (for example at social gatherings, while dancing). It was only through the insight and admission that my passivity had been unnatural that she was brought back to real life, so to speak, as insight does have to reckon with social opposition. Simultaneously it became evident that here again was a case of repetition of the father-child situation. As a child, Dm. had been grossly abused sexually by her father, who was out of control; later, obviously because of the father's bad conscience and social anxiety, he reviled her, so to speak. The daughter had to take revenge on her father indirectly, by failing in her own life.[11]
>
> (Dupont, 1988, pp. 2–3)

In the search for truth, one needs to keep in mind the complexity of the *Clinical Dairy*. An understanding of the subjective workings of any analysis is impossible. Too much happens, much of it is unsaid, and what is said can only possibly be understood within the context of a moment. To understand Thompson's analysis through these *Diary* entries results at best in a fragment of a story. Listening to Thompson about Ferenczi's method is the closest we can come to an understanding of his techniques and to what happened in her analytic treatment. Thompson (1944) argued as much when she said, "Only his pupils, in private conversations, obtained an uncensored glimpse of Ferenczi's own thinking. This thinking deviated quite radically from that outlined in most of his published works" (Thompson, 1944, p. 247). She wrote that his ideas were taught "chiefly by word of mouth through group and individual discussion. This makes it a difficult subject for the historian to pull together" (Thompson, 1944, p. 226). The Diary entry continues:

> The natural behavior of the analyst itself offers points of attack for the opposition. The most extreme consequence of this was drawn by that female patient who demanded that the patient should also have the right to analyze the analyst. In most cases this demand can be met by: (1) admitting in theory to the possibilities of one's own unconscious; (2) relating fragments from one's own past.
>
> It also gave me an opportunity to express ideas and views about the patient that otherwise would not have come to her notice; for example, I could mention utterances indicating moral or aesthetic distaste, an opinion I had heard about her somewhere, etc. If we can teach the patient to cope with all this, we are helping him to cope in general, hastening his release from analysis and the analyst, and we also hasten the transformation into memory of those tendencies toward repetition, hitherto resistant to change.
>
> (p. 3)

The above passage confirms that Ferenczi is modifying Freud's clinical theories; he is developing his own therapeutic methods; and he is moving without pause between talking about Dm. (Thompson) and talking about R.N. (Severn).

12 January 1932
Case of schizophrenia progressive (R.N.)

1. Where the first shock occurred at the age of one and a half years (a promise by an adult, a close relative, to give her something good, instead of which, drugged and sexually abused). At the onset of semiconsciousness, sudden awareness of something vile, total disillusionment and helplessness, perhaps also a temporary feeling of incapacity to exercise her own will, that is, painful awareness of suggestibility . . . At age five renewed,

brutal attack; genitals artificially dilate, insistent suggestion to be compliant with men; stimulating intoxicants administered . . . sudden recollection of the events in the second year of life, suicide impulse, probably also the sensation of dying.

(Dupont, 1988, p. 8)

This is the history of R.N. (Elizabeth Severn), who was brutally abused sexually by her father. Her psychic fragmentation is documented by Ferenczi in the *Clinical Diary* and examined by Rachman (2017), as he discusses her life and her contributions to the psychoanalytic treatment of sexual abuse.

> 17 January 1932
>
> Second case of mutual analysis
>
> The revelation of one's own feelings of anxiety and guilt enables the same tendencies to emerge for the first time in the analysand (Dm.), who in a similar way ruins all potentialities in her life and many of her analyses.
>
> (Dupont, 1988, p. 15)

Since Thompson had only one analytic treatment before Ferenczi, the statement that she "ruins all potentialities in her life and many of her analyses" is more likely about R.N., who had multiple analyses and careers. Ferenczi describes "a slow thawing" with progress toward "trust" in the analysis of a patient that could be either Severn or Thompson. This notation continues:

> One could almost say that the more weaknesses an analyst has, which lead to greater or lesser mistakes and errors but which are then uncovered and treated in the course of mutual analysis, the more likely the analysis is to rest on profound and realistic foundations.
>
> The analysis began years ago, with all possible sternness and reserve, unnecessarily exacerbated by a desire not to allow social differences to interfere. The patient who had come with the intention of opening up in complete freedom, became as though paralyzed, at least in her behavior. Inwardly full of the most intense transference feelings, she did not reveal any of these. A slow thawing, later on definite progress towards trust, particularly when in a moment of great

distress (money matters) she found protection and help from me, and probably also some emotional response. Then came an attempt at displacement onto a third person (R.T.) but, finally, after a second trauma (brother's death), also mitigated by me, she resigned herself to returning to her family and her duties. At this point I succeeded in diverting the patient away from a one-sided (*einseitigen*) interest in ghosts and metaphysics, yet bound up with a great deal of anxiety, to two-sided (*beiderseitigen*) interests (remaining friends with the spirits, but also being able to willing to provide helpful assistance in the real world). What appears to be totally absent is any desire for sexual activity.

(Dupont, 1988, pp. 15–16)

Ferenczi starts out talking about Dm. but then appears to reference someone else, most likely S.I. (Countess Harriot Sigray), whose brother died unexpectedly of a heart attack in November 1930. Thompson's brother, Frank, died in 1997. Thompson may have had some financial problems, as suggested in her letter to Izette De Forest (June 9, 1932), where she points out that only three of her patients were able to pay her (see Brennan, 2015, p. 92, note #11). More likely, however, these notes are a mix-up of patients that include Elizabeth Severn, who was sexually abused, and Countess Harriot Sigray, whose brother died during her treatment.

The 17 January notation then shifts attention:

At this stage the patient begins to show interest and concern for the analyst's psyche. She asks him not to exert himself so desperately; he should not be embarrassed to fall asleep, if he feels like it; thus similar to case no. 1.

(Dupont, 1988, p. 16)

Ferenczi has already referenced case number 1 as a "case of schizophrenia progressive (R.N.)." Thompson and Severn could have both been concerned about Ferenczi's health at this point. As to the lack of sexual interest, Thompson was having an affair with Teddy Miller that year, a confirmation of sorts of her sexual interest. Miller listed Thompson's address as his in his travel papers. This again appears to be a "mix-up of patients."

Mutual Participation

13 March 1932

A "two-children" analysis

Certain phases of mutual analysis represent the complete renunciation of all compulsion and of all authority on both sides: they give the
impression of two equally terrified children who compare their experiences, and because of their common fate understand each other completely and instinctively try to comfort each other.

(Dupont, 1988, p. 56)

A subsection of this notation is titled

Praise necessary:

A patient (Dm.) who for quite a long time has been protesting more or
less unconsciously against the analysis by shifting her love and interest to a young man [Teddy Miller] (probably with the expectation that
I would hate her for it, even if I never said so) one day spontaneously suggests that she will perhaps give up her relationship with this
unsuitable and also much younger man. There upon signs of resistance, which were not resolved until after she had told me how disap-
pointed she was that I did not acknowledge how great a sacrifice she
was making of her own free will. I admitted that she was right. She
then appeared to want to search for the causes of my omission, and we
were able to establish that the patient had been in a state of resistance
for the past three or four months. Cause: the episode of her gossiping
about me, and the consequences for me, namely from Freud, etc. (She
said) I had been more reserved since then, that is, irritable and contemptuous. I had taken the whole thing too personally, instead of looking further for the causes, etc. This was also the cause of the above
omission. The end of the session in a conciliatory mood; she retained
the feeling that she had regained my trust. That I do not treat her as she
had been treated in the past, by her father and also by that teacher, who
never confessed their offenses toward her. Out of revenge, she then
described some of these incidents in much more crude and dreadful
terms than was objectively justified. The hypocrisy of the adults gives

the child justification for exaggerating and lying. If those in authority are more sincere, the child will then come forward on its own with confessions and proposals for good behavior (*mit Vorschlagen zur Gute*). Every such conflict, however, like a quarrel between mother and child, will have to end with reconciliation and praise, that is, signs of trust.

(Dupont, 1988, p. 57)

This notation is a coherent explanation of what possibly went on between Thompson and Ferenczi. It is a rare look at the process in their treatment. It begins with Ferenczi having withdrawn from Thompson following her telling Edith Jackson she kissed him and Freud's ensuing reprimand. Ferenczi is "irritable and contemptuous" toward her. She is resisting his efforts to get her to end her relationship with Teddy Miller. At first, they both attribute her "resistance" to her affair with Miller. She agrees to give up the relationship for the treatment and expects Ferenczi to acknowledge her sacrifice. What Ferenczi does not accept is that Thompson provoked him knowingly. Instead, he reduces her provocation to "gossip," a type of objectification of female communication. Thompson, on the other hand, wants him to look more deeply into his feelings toward her. She felt he was avoiding examining what had occurred. He felt she found relief in his disclosures and experienced being treated differently by him than she was by her father and most likely her teacher, Adolf Meyer. What also appears here is the notion that she lied and/or exaggerated, out of revenge, about both her father and Meyer. Did Thompson lie about her father? Did her father turn against her in the way that Adolf Meyer ceased to support her? We know that Meyer did not admit his anger toward her for abandoning him, it appears her father did not admit his abandonment of her either.

Ferenczi suggests that Thompson lied or exaggerated something about her father and her teacher. He feels that hypocrisy in adults gives the child/patient justification for lying. He finds adult/therapist honesty begets child/patient honesty.

Toward a Theory of the Defensive Use of Smell

Ferenczi's interest with odor occupies many months of notations in the *Clinical Diary*. He was working on an understanding the use of odor as a defensive (see pgs. 86–131). These notations might be an example of Clara Thompson's (1944) observation that Ferenczi tended to carry his ideas to extremes. It is in the following notations that we learn of Thompson's abuse at the hands of her mother.

24 April 1932

Paranoia and the sense of smell

A patient reports that on the previous day she had to spend several hours in the company of Mrs. (sic) Dm., a lady she had known for quite some time, and who had also made several attempts at analytic treatment with her. The reasons she gave for her antipathy toward this lady were her lack of education, her New England narrow-mindedness, and her primitive way of expressing herself; furthermore, she did not have the least trace of artistic elan, etc. This prompted her to flee from the company of this lady. As she could not avoid her yesterday, she felt compelled to get drunk. Only in a totally drunk, unbalanced, dreamy, half-asleep state could she stand her. When thinking of her, all her associations centered on the smell of this lady. She gives off an odor like that of a corpse, which scares the patient and alerts her defenses.

On the same day Dm. came to see me and said that she had also drunk a lot (but had not been drunk). She feels frightened in the company of the patient; this lady, she said, was too aggressive, too energetic, and reminded her of her own mother. (Here the link with an infantile trauma: her mother had grabbed her so hard by the wrist that she broke her arm.) It must be noted here that Dm. does really have a very unpleasant odor, and people with a fairly acute sense of smell definitely are repelled by her. It may be stated as highly probable that the intensity of these emanations may have something to do with repressed hate and rage. It is as if, like certain animals, in the absence of other available weapons she keeps people away from her body with such repellent emanations of hate. (Consciously and in her manifest behavior, the patient is rather pliant and inclined to blind obedience and uncomplaining submissiveness.)

. . . It was not too presumptuous to trace the patient's [Elizabeth Severn's?] reaction to the fact that she can actually smell people's feelings. She also reported then to me various other experiences of this kind. Interestingly, she gives me a long account of her mother, who had concocted for herself ideas similar to those of Professor Jaeger in his time. Having a bath and washing were unhealthy, she never changed her underwear, but she felt she never had an unpleasant smell. Otherwise she was uncommonly energetic and ruled in the home (the father was a drunk, and only entered the house once in a while, soon after which another child would be born).

The theory that could be derived from these and similar questions would be as follows: The emanations of the patient's mother, which were consciously aggressive, did not stink, yet those of Dm., who was seemingly more obsequious and accommodating, but secretly is filled with hate, betray this repressed hatred (here the association "Solomon the Wise speaks?).""

These passages switch from R.N. to Dm. One wonders could Thompson have emitted such an offensive odor. To do so, she would have had to fall far from her roots of hygiene and dress as a well-schooled Pembroke girl. Interviews with people who knew her all agreed she was always clean and there was never a hint of a bad odor.

Ferenczi continues to note the defensive operations of odor:

Dm. is frightened by the openly aggressive manner of the patient [most likely Elizabeth Severn] and begins to stink. The patient [Elizabeth Severn] perceives this as a counterattack, as being persecuted (persecution mania), and must either run away or anesthetize herself with alcohol. It is not impossible that in so doing she is imitating her father, an alcoholic, who could not stand to be with her mother. As long as she is manically aggressive, she imitates her mother; however, when she begins to sense Dm.'s hidden aggression, she then begins to play the role of the father (?). Be that as it may in detail, this much is certain, that those suffering from persecution mania—like certain animals, especially dogs—can smell people's hidden or repressed emotions and tendencies. A further step would lead to an extraordinarily more subtle and more finely gradated qualitative and quantitative sensibility that would enable someone to smell the most delicate emotions and even the psychic content of wishful impulses, that is, the representations of another person. A great deal of what has been regarded up to now as occult, or as a metaphysical superperformance, would thus become explicable in psychophysicological terms. A further and still bolder step would then lead to total emanations, as they continue vibrating somewhere in space, even across the limitless passage of the ages. (As a dog might [sense] the footprints of its deceased master.) Spiritualist mediums, therefore, reconstruct, with the aid of their sense of smell, a person's past. They may, aided by their olfactory imagination, follow a person back into the most distant past, to all the places he stayed in the course of his life.

Why Dm.'s smell should be experienced as the smell of a corpse is a problem in itself. A preliminary attempt at a solution: whenever an emotional reaction is suppressed, interrupted, or repressed, something is actually destroyed in us. The annihilated part of the person falls into a state of decay and decomposition. Should the entire person be prevented from acting, then generalized decomposition ensures, that is to say, death. A link here with the assertion has so many neurotics, in states of trance or dream states, that a, greater or less or part of them is dead, or killed, and is dragged around, as a lifeless, that is, nonfunctioning burden. The content of this burden of repression is in a permanent state of agony, that is, decomposition. Total disintegration (death) is just as impossible for it as coming back to life through the influx of vital energies.

Nine pin.

Silly servant.

(Dupont, 1988, pp. 86–88)

Ferenczi is trying to explain the corpse like smell in terms of Dm.'s repressed and decaying feelings rather than analyzing Severn's association to a corpse based on her early history. A corpse had particular significance for Ferenczi, one appeared in his dream. Severn too had an experience with a corpse, she was shown a corpse when she was a child. But these events do not work their way into Ferenczi's conscious associations. Instead, Thompson's "odor" is his focus. One might wonder, did she use deodorant? As she became more anxious, did her perspiration increase, or did she use a cover-up cologne, as many people did at that time, that emitted a fragrance that Ferenczi and Severn both found offensive?

Could Ferenczi's concerns with odor be related to his sexual abuse as a child?[12]

Ways of Being Passionate, Power, and the Death Drive

There are five separate entries dated June 3, 1932.

3 June 1932
Theoretical consequences for libido-theory and neurosis-theory
Symptomatology of infantile sexuality must be differentiated more precisely than before into (a) spontaneous and (b) provoked excitation . . . (Adults should know that they cannot count on the child's gratitude.) . . . ("one is one's own mother, in fact the mother of the mother.") Capacity for guiltless enjoyment . . . Adjustment to reality through one's own experience . . .

(Dupont, 1988, p. 113)

3 June 1932
No special training analysis!
analysts should be analyzed *better, not worse*, than patients . . . mutual analysis only a last resort! Proper analysis by a stranger, without any obligation, would be better . . . The best analyst is a patient who has been cured . . . Doubts about *supervised analyses:* last resorts: recognition and admission of one's own difficulties and weaknesses. Strictly supervised by the patients! No attempts to defend oneself. (p. 115)

The third notation speaks to Dm. and her ways of being passionate:

3 June 1932
(Dm.) Ways of being passionate. Concluded.
Symptom: *Buying* oneself *peace* and *friendliness* by excessive expenditure of tenderness and presents of money. Fear that without these one will remain alone. Better to give away everything. Behind this: outbursts of rage if the *most exaggerated* expectation of pleasure without reciprocity is not fulfilled by every object, every person. First impulse: to destroy the unaccommodating world! Then becoming aware of *anxiety, obedience exaggerated*, solely in order to escape the anxiety. (p. 115)

Ferenczi then asks:
Is not anxiety therefore in the last analysis, a feeling of the power of the death drive, a beginning of death (starvation)?

Dm. (1) was born with teeth, the same as her brother, that is, with the strongest aggressive tendencies. (2) Breast refused. Bottle. When she asserted herself: mother like ice.

Indifference, (2) aggression, (3) excessive tenderness: all three have a regressive effect on the child. The child senses, correctly, the aggressive element even in exaggerated libidinal passion. (Transient symptom on this point: she feels smothered. (p. 115)

Did Thompson attempt to purchase peace and friendliness with expressions of tenderness? Was she prone to giving literal gifts to buy the affection of others? Was she afraid of being alone or unloved? Did she become enraged when her expectations for love were not fulfilled? It is unclear when Ferenczi writes "Concluded" if he is indicating that the patient stopped these defensive ways of being.

These notations confirm again that Thompson's mother was cold. The young Thompson's attempts at self-assertion were met with maternal indifference or, worse, aggression or fake displays of tenderness. In the process of understanding this in her treatment, she may at times felt smothered.

3 June 1932

Passion

. . . TO KILL. Which is primary: aggressiveness, or regression to self-destruction? . . . THERAPY . . . Analysis must make possible for the patient, morally and physically, the *utmost regression*, without shame! Only then will the patient, after he (or she) has enjoyed for a while taking everything for nothing without scruples of conscience, be able to adapt to the facts; even to tolerate maternally (without expecting anything in return) the sufferings of others (goodness) is about passion and an exaggeration of obedience. (p. 116)

These are important comments on the process of analysis that hint at infant and caregiver patterns of affect regulation. Contemporary infant research indicates "the child's developmental process should be assessed by the degree to which patterns of affect regulation remain warm and mutual" (Beebe & Lachmann, 2002, p. 16).

(Dm.) There is no goodness where gratitude is expected. One should have received kindness as a child, and so much of it that one can pass some of it on (to the next generation). (Mention Dm!)

Obedient children of passionate parents have to be cleverer than their parents, play a maternal role.

(My own experience: mother in a rage.)

Passion: *incestuous relation*: for the child it is only aggression.

(B.) Icy coldness—sensed in Mrs. E. [unknown person] Her own feelings: (1) Compulsion to soften that coldness by means of exaggerated amiability. (2) Behind this the feeling: (a) I do not love her, I do not love anyone (friendly toward everybody). Obviously, I expect to be loved by everybody. (b) Anger because this does not happen. Aggressiveness provoked and intensified to the point of wanting to kill. (c) Fear of being alone, of not being loved. The condition of being loved must be attained, in any circumstances. (d) This happens in an exaggerated way. (pp. 116–117)

These are continuous process notes that reflect either five sessions in one day or five thoughts about the session on the third of June. The theme is consistent. A synopsis might look something like this. How does a young child get love? Thompson wanted love from her analyst, love she should have received from her mother (parents). She tried to be an obedient child and in the process learned how to manage her parents (becoming the parent). That strategy worked to some degree, but it left her feeling enraged. In her regressed state with her analyst, she met a parental figure who was not abusive or rejecting, but he is imperfect. They struggle human to human, and she emerges with a better sense of herself.

There are four entries under the date June 12, 1932. One of them cites Dm.

12 June 1932

Failures with pupils

. . . Dm. now has the courage to reproach me for abandoning pupils at the first signs of incomplete adaptation or submission. I have to admit to it, but excuse myself with the argument that pupils do steal my ideas without quoting me. Freud has found the same symptom in my brother complex, which has recurred now in the International Association. (p. 122)

Thompson reproached Ferenczi for abandoning a patient too early. He admits he gives up and defends himself with an argument that pupils steal his ideas without quoting him. By this time, Thompson has published her essay " 'Dutiful Child' Resistance," (1931) a paper that addresses the themes that have surfaced in her analysis.

The entry, dated June 14, 1932, includes two notations. The first has to do with patient (U), Theodore (Teddy) Miller, the man with whom Thompson was having an intimate relationship.

14 June 1932

Permanent disturbance of object-libido

1. Patient U. notices in himself that he feels no inclination for preliminary pleasure or foreplay in sexual relations, but experiences the act more like an obligation, as it were, which he seeks to get over as quickly possible, similar lack of "after pleasure" [*Nachlust*]. He is puzzled when he hears from one of his mistresses that she is "thrilled" for quite some time both before and after. Explanation: a young savage, raised in the most primitive circumstances, suddenly arrives at the age of twelve in an environment that, at least on the surface, is far more civilized (emigration to America). At first degraded in his entire personality, he uses psychoanalysis as a springboard to rise to a more sublimated sphere (in order to rid himself of his perpetual fear; fear of going mad). A more recent breakdown during a first analysis, when in bad company he is threatened with death . . . He does not believe in subtleties, tenderness, symbolism, allusions, moral inhibitions, etc., only direct action itself seems real to him. He battles against his own criminal and ruthlessly infantile-egoistic tendencies . . . it is also possible that some kind of homosexual experiences caused him to turn away from the female sex. II. Patient O.S.: Infantile traumata: (1) anal injury caused in two different ways, by a woman and a man . . . III. Latent feelings of hatred, overt friendliness and kindness, anal fissure, conspicuously smelly emanations. Principal motive for these tendencies of hatred and superiority stems from the conviction that as a child she was deceived and defeated in the struggle for her father's love. The father only played with her, it was the mother who had the baby. Since then no tender love relationship, even the present one is bound up with hatred, largely anal (independent) and strongly aggressive. (pp. 122–124)

Thompson did not want Ferenczi to give up on patient U. (Teddy Miller). Ferenczi notes how U. "felt no pleasure in sexual relations" and how he "does not believe in subtleties, tenderness etc." Ferenczi wanted Thompson to stop seeing Miller, and she said she did (see Ferenczi, 1949b).

After Ferenczi's death, Thompson wrote to her friend Ilona Vass (letter quoted in Shapiro, 1993, p. 168),

> Yes, I feel now that I can stand alone without support. For a long time after Dr. Ferenczi died, I clung to Teddy and he to me, but gradually it became apparent that one of us must get free because we were in a way holding each other down.

This letter confirms that although she told Ferenczi she ended her relationship with Miller, their attachment continued. She goes on to say,

> So I have done a lot of self analysis this winter and I think that I am today better than I ever was in my life. I do not say that my life is solved exactly as I would have it solved if there were a good fairy somewhere who would give me just what I want. But perhaps it is solved as well as it can be. Anyway I don't feel I have reached the limit of my development yet. I am going next week to spend part of my vacation with my mother. I could never have wanted to do that before and now I rather look forward to it. I have had some nice times with men this winter too. It seems that I have lost my contempt for them and I used to have contempt similar to your own.
>
> (8/3/34)

The second entry on June 14, 1932, begins a discussion about feminism and homosexuality. Thompson, along with her friends Alice Lowell and Izette de Forest, talk with Ferenczi about their sexuality and feminist ideas.

14 June 1932

Normalis feminin homosexualitas

"Men don't understand," women say, and are (even in analysis) very reticent about their feelings. "men think women can only love the possessors of penises." In reality, they continue to long for a mother and female friend, with whom they can talk about their heterosexual experiences—without jealousy. (B, and Ett., Dm. and women friends). They prefer effeminate (passive, homosexual) men, because these offer them a continuation of bisexuality.

(Dupont, 1988, pp. 124–125)

The renunciation of homosexuality

(Repression occurs at the time of first menstruation—when Tom-Boy-ishness is suppressed all of a sudden.) Dm. demands from me (after overcoming substantial resistance) *that I should become a good mother to U (and to herself)*

[Here there is a footnote explaining that Ferenczi is discussing his relationships to U., a man, and Dm., a woman.]

(Dm.): I am to overcome my ambition to be greater than he, content myself with a passive role in relation to him, but at the same time also accept her tomboy-love. Only then will she permit herself to cut herself loose from her dependence on me. Masculine or feminine: I must admit that I *love* U. (Daddy!) *just as much as I love her* then we (daughter and mother) will become colleagues. A large share of the girl's *tenderness* remains (under such circumstances) attached to the mother. (p. 125)

Thompson's bisexuality is mentioned here as it was in an interview with her friend Zeborah Schachtel. Thompson had lifelong relationships with Lowell and de Forest, who acknowledged their sexual relationship; Lowell appears to have been an out lesbian during this period. Was Thompson involved with either of them romantically? There are references by Ferenczi to her "tom-boy love" in this section. Those are his words, not Thompson's. Shapiro (1993) lends some support for her bisexuality citing a letter to Maurice Green from Edith Sprague Field (fn. p. 165) where she notes, "her [Thompson's] life at college triggered the first of several rumors of lesbian relationships."

That Thompson would wish for Ferenczi to be a "good mother" to her boyfriend Teddy seems consistent with what we know about her caring attitude toward others. She wanted Ferenczi to take care of Miller to free her from that responsibility (see below a discussion in "Notes and Fragments"). At that point, she wanted to be Ferenczi's colleague, since no doubt she was his collaborator. However, Ferenczi has a hard time disentangling himself from the Freudian oedipal concept. He arrives at the feeling that he must become a mother to Thompson. In doing so, he offers her tenderness, affection, and empathy, the qualities missing from her relationship with her mother.

More on Odor as a Defense

19 June 1932

Specific odor of the mentally ill

. . . Patient Dm., who herself in fact perspires quite conspicuously and with a marked odor, particularly on certain occasions, finds a similarity between herself and the mentally ill Mrs. Smith. (I had an opportunity to see Mrs. Smith, a schizophrenic, in a state of terrible anxiety. She did have a penetrating smell, rather like mouse urine.)

Dm., on the other hand, feels that she herself exudes sexual odors. She also suffers from anal fissure. Both conditions, as well as intermittently chronic contractions, become manifest when she suppresses her tendency toward almost manic rage in speech, voice, and gestures. The suppressed rage stimulates a chemical change in her (poisoning—see poison for rage), the transformation of the attracting substance into one that repels. The analysis reveals that she is waiting for a hero, who will not be scared off even by the odors. The analyst must be this hero, he must (1) abandon his hypocritical insensitivity and admit his antipathy and his revulsion; (2) analyze himself, or let himself be analyzed to a point where he no longer finds such substances and behavior repellent, whereupon (3) the patient will renounce her provocative activities.

In the case of Dm., acquaintance with the analyst began with the patient behaving quite improperly at a dance. After she was not accepted as a patient at that time, she went straight to the apartment of a young man and lost her virginity. Naturally this provoked reactions of disgust in the analyst, which had to be overcome in the course of a prolonged period of work.

The model for this whole process was infantile rage concerning (1) the prohibition of all sexual expressions, (2) the realization that the parents engaged in sexual activities (birth of children). A further motive to fury was anger over the weak submission of the father to the maternal power (some of what appears as penis envy may be a demonstration of the behavior of a woman who remained with a weak man).

(Dupont, 1988, pp. 131–132)

There are many points that stand out in this notation sequence:

We learn that patient Dm. perspires with a marked odor; she feels she exudes sexual odors from her genitals; she suffers from an anal fissure. Do these odors intensify when she becomes angry or anxious? There is a switch to the topic of mutual analysis that alerts the reader to Elizabeth Severn who may again be mixed up with Thompson. The note, "a tendency to almost manic rage in speech voice and gestures" does not sound like Thompson but could be Severn.

Did Thompson have sex for the first time as an act of revenge against Ferenczi because he did not take her on as an analysand in New York? She could also have felt better about herself for approaching Ferenczi and freed up enough to have a sexual encounter. Why would Ferenczi react with "disgust" over her behavior? Did he think it improper for her to have a sexual life? What does it mean to behave improperly at a dance? Was she overly seductive with him? With someone else? We can't know the answers to these questions and again it could be a mix up of patients.

What do we know? Patient Dm. perspires, she has an anal fissure which could be the source of an odor and, she worries about having a sexual odor. In Thompson's (1950b) "Some effects of the derogatory attitude toward female sexuality," she focuses on societal attitudes toward female genitals and the excessive emphasis on "cleanliness," noting how it affects a women's sense of self. She gives us examples of a patient who was troubled because she felt her body "stinking." This could be autobiographical. She speaks of a situation where "the mother was cold and puritanical as well as overclean. The patient felt humiliated because she had a healthy sexual drive which she felt was made known to the world by her body's odors and secretions" (p. 354). These biased cultural attitudes toward women not only saturate and complicate these notations but they most likely were Thompson's personal concerns.

Ferenczi's references to the "prohibition of all sexual expression," and "A further motive to fury was anger over the weak submission of the father to the maternal power (some of what appears as penis envy may be a demonstration of the behavior of a woman who remained with a weak man)" is a repeating refrain in Dm.'s treatment.

Motives for Penis Envy

20 June 1932

Another motive for women's wish to have a penis

The principal motive in Dm.; the desire to be loved by her mother. "Mother always found something wrong with her body" (even in her

earliest childhood, criticizing her chubbiness, her odor (?)—her passionate way of hugging, even more, *her love for her father*, which was
passionate at an early age). Her desire to become a boy was determined
by the wish to eliminate her mother's *dislike of her feminine inclina-
tions*. She disguises herself as a man *because as a woman she dis-
pleases her mother* (is hated by her mother, very likely for reasons of
jealousy). This wish intensifies at the onset of *puberty*, when femininity
can no longer be denied. (Menstruation.) She is aware that her mother
is displeased (envy, jealousy). She seeks out masculine activities. She
feels that her mother will not let her *really* get married and obeys her; or
that her mother looks for quite unsuitable men for her. When she herself
falls in love with someone (father, B.[Alice Lowell] Mac.), it ends in
tragedy. She wants (dream fantasy) to be loved by the analyst, despite
another man's passion and moods.

Yet equally, she wants only a man who recognizes that a woman
has other desires beyond genital gratification—Which only a mother is
capable of satisfying. *Longing for a triangle without envy or jealousy.*

(Dupont, 1988, p. 132)

Thompson's wish to be physically accepted by Ferenczi (the kiss) becomes
understandable given her early deprivation of affection. Becoming a physician was thought of then as a "masculine activity." Could the wished-for
triangle in this discussion be between de Forest, Lowell, and Thompson?
The statement that "a woman has other desires beyond genital gratification" could be heard as a feminist position.

There are two notations on June 24, 1932:

24 June 1932 [1]
  On failing to hear (Vom Uberhoren). A specific form of parapraxis
  Actors: Dm. Mrs. Sp. Mrs Sch.
  A B C
  A, B, C sunbathing together.
  Account of the events by AB and BC:
  The three of them talked together for quite a while; finally Dm.
takes her leave. B. [Lowell] and C.[Mrs. Sch.] under the impression
that A [Dm.] has already gone, C in particular starts to malign her,
quite openly, even in a loud voice. She is "common." Her language
low—scum of populace. No originality, boring, common, common,

common.—Suddenly appears Dm. who after taking leave had sat down in nearby bathing hut, arranging her hair. "Now I caught you," she said, and departed with an angry expression. (Even that was "common," said C. She, C, would have done it differently, with more finesse.) In any case, B and C are greatly disturbed over the incident. (p. 143)

Account by A (all this in analysis) [Dm.]

"I had an epileptic fit." Yesterday Gellert Swimming Pool—then Pest—then home in bed. Jerks for hours. Not a word about the incident! Because I suspected an intentional failure to hear, I told her the story of B. and C. She knows nothing about it; she was not listening.

Theory: 1. She heard everything

2. Aided by her capacity to *swallow* the most unjust accusations, she swallows the knowledge of what she has heard. *She fails to hear* nonsense, lies, and injustice—in order not to explode (kill).

3. All previous outranges of such a kind return and cause (a) an unconscious range ("epileptic fit"), (b) dreams with references to the word not heard and to its associations (mother, I). Seemingly senseless emotions, *outbursts,* and *movements* are revealed as unconscious range and reactions of revenge. (c) connection between parapraxis and dream. Dream of the following night contains a reference to the incident and the history of its origin.

The process of repression

1. *Onset* of a reaction.

2. Change of direction in the *statu nascendi* (perhaps imaginary identification with the aggressor) or "taking him ad absurdum," in the hope that he will finally realize this. (?) In any event: splitting off of the emotion. Reaction in *the body of ego consciousness (Ichbewusstsein).* Leap into the physical sphere of the body. Originally every reaction bodily and psychic. From now on: ability to *react with the body alone.*

(Dupont, 1988, p. 143)

24 June 1932 [2]

Yesterday, she reports, she was in a bad mood . . . She read two chapters of Chadwick's book; yesterday she thought she had read in this book the idea about anxiety and a feeling of filthiness (leakage) accompanying menstruation . . . *On second reading* it now becomes evident (the truth!) that Chadwick had written nothing about it. She wanted to make a present to Chadwick of her own idea (unconsciously) . . . C.

recounts a dream of the same night:. . . trauma (a) caused by a man is true: mother's doubts make the child consciously deny her own self . . . (pp. 144–145)

It is not clear who Ferenczi is discussing. The only initial given is C. Perhaps he is referring to the C in the Gellert pool episode. There are two June 30, 1932, entries. The first one is unique in that Ferenczi refers to "Dr. Thompson" rather than using the initials Dm. He then identifies a line from a paper she wrote: "at the beginning of life people have no individuality." Ferenczi goes on to discuss the projection of adult psychology onto children as an intrapsychic process. The second entry is about hypocrisy and the theme of how adults who lie to children create deceptive children.

30 June 1932
Projection of adult psychology onto children (falsum)
It is certain that Freud has succeeded in tracing the psychology of the adult genetically far back into childhood. Starting with the assumption that the reactions of children, babies, indeed all living beings are identical with those of adults, the difference being that children are prevented from asserting their original longings for omnipotence, which they retain secretly in a repressed form for the rest of their lives . . . In one psychic process the importance of which has perhaps been insufficiently appreciated, even by Freud himself, namely that of identification as a stage preceding object relations, we have until recently not sufficiently appreciated the functioning in it of a mode of reaction already lost to us, but one that nevertheless exists . . . a different kind of reaction principle . . . a state in which any act of self-protection or defense is excluded and all external influence remains an impression without any internal anti-cathexis . . . The most concise summary of this situation was perhaps given by Dr. Thompson, when she said that people at the beginning of their lives have as yet no individuality. Here my view on the tendency to fade away (falling ill and dying in very young children) and the predominance in them of the death instinct; their extreme impressionability (mimicry) may be also just a sign of rather weak life and self assertive instincts;. . . The hallucitory period . . . is preceded by a purely mimetic period . . . protection is the original form of life. (p. 148)

30 June 1932

Hypocrisy and the "enfant terrible"

Dm: hypocrisy is the consequence of cowardice in those who set the tone. (Authorities are afraid of authorities.) They preach lying and speak contemptuously of anyone who speaks the unadorned truth. *Good children* have become hypocrites themselves. "Enfants terribles" are in revolt (perhaps to an extreme) against hypocrites and exaggerate simplicity and democracy. Really favorable development (optimum) would lead to the development of individuals (and a race) that would be neither mendacious (hypocritical) nor destructive.

Schizophrenia is a "photochemical" mimicry reaction, instead of self-assertion (revenge defense). (Dm: schizophrenics were affected by trauma *before* they possessed a personality.) . . . *Influence of the passions of adults on the character-neuroses and sexual development of children* [An editorial footnote indicates that this passage contains an outline of the ideas that Ferenczi presented at the congress of Wiesbaden in 1932 in "The Confusion of Tongues between Adults and the Child."]

What are passions? . . . The fact of *feeling-one's self* postulates the existence of a *non-I; the ego is an abstraction*. PRIOR to this abstraction we must have felt the Whole (universe).

The child is still closer to this feeling of universality (without sense organs), he knows (feels) everything, certainly much more than adults, whose present sense organs serve in large part to exclude a large part of the external world (in fact *everything* except what is useful).

Adults are relative idio`ts. Children are all knowing. (pp. 149–150)

The next notation is a continuation of the ideas presented in the "Confusion of Tongues" paper.

6 July 1932

Projection of our own passions or passionate tendencies onto children

Are perversions really infantilisms, and to what extent? Are sadism and anal eroticism not already hysterical reactions to traumata? . . . if one goes too thoroughly into the positive or negative countertransference, one may avoid unpleasant experiences in the course of the sessions, but if one does not evade it, then one may be rewarded by unexpected progress.

Dm.: Ever since she sees and feels that I do not respond to her provocative actions and behavior simply with antipathy, one can have anything from her. There is enormous progress. (pp. 155–157)

And next:

19 July 1932
Superiority (grandeur) up to now has given me the pleasant feeling that everyone is stupid (crazy) but me. Psychoanalytical insight into my own emotional emptiness, which was shrouded by overcompensation (repressed—unconscious—psychosis) led to a self-diagnosis of schizophrenia. (In consequence, compensations had to be in conflict with reality, that is, delusional, paranoid. Hatred of the woman, veneration of man (with a compulsion to promiscuity as a superstructure) made possible the rationalization of traumatic impotence . . . In Cases II, IV. (Dm., B., etc.,) faster (pp. 159–161)

The July 24, 1932, entry is a discussion of various patients. He is still working on ideas in the "Confusion of Tongues" paper, including the essence of the paper:

the adaptive potential "response" of even very young children to sexual or other passionate attacks is much greater than one would imagine. Traumatic confusion arises mainly because the attack and the response to it are denied by the guilt-ridden adults, indeed, are treated as deserving punishment.

(p. 178)

It is not until page 172 that he notates something about Dm:

24 July 1932
    Identification versus hatred
    1. G. Mother = father. Left alone.
2. Dm.—No comparison with unprovocative, reasonable people, as their existence is unknown. The child sees parents fighting (senseless, mad). If I admit this then I am left without parents; that is, however (for a child), absolutely impossible. Therefore the child becomes a psychiatrist, who treats the madman with understanding and tells him that he is right (This way he will be less dangerous.) Indeed, the child even

commits mistakes on purpose in order to justify and satisfy the adults' need for aggression.

(Dm.: smelling.) (p. 172)

From late July to early October, there are no direct references to Dm. Ferenczi returns to the issue of mutuality in early October, proclaiming mutuality as an essential ingredient in treatment.

2 October 1932

Mutuality—sine qua

An attempt to continue analyzing unilaterally. Emotionality disappeared; analysis insipid. Relationship—distant. Once mutuality has been attempted, one-sided analysis then is no longer possible—not productive.

Now the question: must every case be mutual?—and to what extent?

1. U.: Confession of weakness had made him anxious—helpless—contemptuous.

2. Dm.: Made herself independent—feels hurt because of the absence of mutuality on my part. At the same time, she becomes convinced that she has overestimated father's (and my) importance. Everything comes from the mother. (pp. 213–214)

In this last notation in the Clinical *Diary*, Ferenczi wonders if every case needs to be a mutual analysis. He notes that Thompson has made herself "independent," though she feels "hurt" that he did not pursue his "mutuality" with her in the same way he did with other patients. The most meaningful line in the notation may be that at the end of her analysis, Thompson was convinced she "overestimated her father's and Ferenczi's importance," concluding instead, "Everything comes from the mother." That conclusion places the notion of sexual abuse by her father again in question, unless she found her mother's coldness and rejection more destructive to her than she did the alleged sexual abuse.

The Deep Freeze

After Ferenczi's death, Judith Dupont, Vilma Kovacs, and Alice Balint advised Mrs. Ferenczi not to publish the notations of the *Clinical Diary* for the "time being." As stated, their thinking was to wait until the "repercussions" of the dispute between Freud and Ferenczi settled down and a more favorable atmosphere developed. While work continued in terms of organizing and translating the material, the second world war interfered with their progress. Freud was reportedly aware of the material and "expressed admiration for Ferenczi's ideas" (Dupont, 1988, p. 219).

Then in 1957, Jones published a "violent attack" on Ferenczi (Dupont, 1988, p. 220). The decision was made again to postpone publishing the *Diary*. It was with the publication of the Freud and Ferenczi correspondence that the Editor, Judith Dupont, and translators thought it the right time to also publish the *Clinical Diary*.

Notes and Fragments: Supplemental Information

However, in 1949, long before the publication of the Clinical Diary, other notes were found among Ferenczi's papers, published as "Notes and Fragments (1930–1932)," and subsequently as the *Final Contributions*. These notes mention Clara Thompson and Teddy Miller. Ferenczi (1949b) writes:

DM. has always had the compulsion to seduce men and to be thrown into disaster by them. In fact she has done so only to escape from the loneliness which was brought upon her by her mother's coldness. Even in the over passionate ruthless expressions of love by her mother, she felt her mother's hatred as a disturbing element (difficult birth, although no actual contraction of the pelvis).
  (p. 233)

PATIENT DM.: Sudden crying when preparing a dinner for U. Has never given up *playing*. She wanted only to play at cooking but was compelled to bear real burdens which were much too difficult.—(Sex!)—Effort to *identification*.)— *Suggestion without analysis = superimposing the hypnotist's superego*. (Over exertion.)—Correct therapy: (*a*) return to childhood—permission to give full vent, (*b*) waiting for the *spontaneous* tendency of "growth,"—here then encouragement certainly has its right place.—Courage must be suggested. Spontaneous *tendency to grow* emerges when play can no longer satisfy the present quantum of energy. (Physical and mental organs develop and demand to be used.)
  (p. 240)

> (Patients Dm., G,) compulsion to solve even the most difficult
> problems.

PATIENT DM.: Fixation to: mother, forcibly dissolved *much too early*.
Compulsion and *overflow*. (p. 239)

These final entries shed additional light on Thompson's struggles with
gender prescriptions and expectations. Her relationship with Teddy Miller
was an effort to escape loneliness. Again, we hear about the destructive-
ness of her mother's coldness. What did Thompson think about her analysis with Ferenczi? She found it to be nearly 100% helpful (see Eissler
interview, chapter one).

Unresolved Issues or Misunderstandings?

Was Clara Thompson the victim of childhood sexual abuse? Are signs of
unresolved issues around abuse apparent in Thompson's behavior? There
is compelling evidence that the patients in the Diary have been voluntarily mixed up to preserve their identity. And there is evidence from Clara
Thompson that explains how she felt misunderstood. For example, in her
letter to Adolf Meyer (Thompson (1926), Adolf Meyer Collection 1890–
1940), she attributes her fall-out with him to his anger with her over her
move toward psychoanalysis, a method of treatment he did not advocate at
the clinic. Thompson was strongly resistant to dogmatic rules and refused
to conform or be intimidated. This interpretation of her behavior is consistent with her character and supported by her wish, to be a woman who
could not be dominated (Interview with Zeborah Schachtel, 2017).

Thompson's mother's physical abuse and critical attitude toward her was
traumatic. She understood that feelings can be transmitted non-verbally
causing confusion and that confusion is part of the presentation of traumatized patients. She disagreed with the practice of encouraging the reliving
of extreme emotions through regression, arguing instead that those feelings would emerge "unwittingly" (Thompson, 1944, p. 251).

What made for a successful analysis? Thompson (1944) reported that
"Ferenczi, at the end of his investigations, is concerned less with the neurotic adult than with the traumatized child present in the adult on the couch,"
and that one of his "greatest assets was his respect for and belief in the
patient" (p. 246). She pointed out that while Freud believed that a child's
struggle with their instincts created their problems, Ferenczi believed the

child became ill as a result of "bad parents" (p. 246). Thompson was critical of Ferenczi's too-intrusive experimental method that pushed for the
patient to relive a traumatic event. She felt that put an unnecessary burden
on the patient. She also thought that he held a limited understanding of the
need for love in treatment. She did not believe an analyst could give the
patient all the love they missed out on in childhood. Instead, she argued
that given the absence of love as a child, when it was given to them as an
adult, it was hard to digest.

In her analysis with Fromm, she refined her understanding of love as the
need to free oneself from the coercion of conformity.[13]

Another Look: Kissing Papa Ferenczi

Clara Thompson appears on page two of the Ferenczi's *Diary* (see Chapter 4) as the first patient to be noted by name and memorialized for kissing
her analyst. Why, of all the unorthodox triangles and enactments that we
have reviewed, is Thompson's confidentiality sacrificed? And why is her
affectionate kiss of Ferenczi deserving of such close attention? According
to Dupont (1995), Ferenczi crossed the patient/therapist boundary when
he spontaneously kissed his patient and later stepdaughter, Elma Palos-
Laurvik and professed his love for her. The details of that encounter are
described in a 1966 letter from Elma Palos-Laurvik to Michael Balint.
Elma wrote Balint:

> I don't want it to harm Sándor's reputation . . . I don't want his oppo-
> nents to find there new opportunities to declare him irresponsible . . .
> I was a young girl of vivid temperament . . . Sándor got up from his
> chair behind me, sat down near me on the couch and, obviously car-
> ried along by passion, kissed me and in a state of great excitement told
> me how much he was in love with me and asked me if I could love
> him. I don't know if it was true or not, but I answered him "yes" and
> I hope that I really believed it . . . I don't remember for how many
> days or weeks Sándor came daily to lunch with us as my fiancé, before
> I realized that already I loved him less than I had thought during the
> analysis . . . Anyway, the whole family situation must have been poi-
> sonous. If I remember well, it is after this event that I went to Vienna
> and was analyzed by Freud for six months . . . When I came back
> to Budapest, Mother and Sándor were already married. When I met

Sándor again for the first time, we both were somewhat embarrassed; but with time passing, the situation became normal.

(p. 829)

How do we understand the motivation and aftermath of Thompson telling Edith Jackson she kissed Ferenczi? In considering motivation, Ferenczi's note directs our attention to her mother:

> The principal motive in Dm.; the desire to be loved by her mother. "Mother always found something wrong with her body" (even in her earliest childhood, criticizing her chubbiness, her odor (?)—her passionate way of hugging, even more, *her love for her father*, which was passionate at an early age). Her desire to become a boy was determined by the wish to eliminate her mother's *dislike of her feminine inclinations*. She disguises herself as a man *because as a woman she displeases her mother* (is hated by her mother, very likely for reasons of jealousy).

> (Dupont, 1988, p. 132)

This excerpt is critical to understanding Clara Thompson. It is about being abused by her mother, not her father. Ferenczi offered to create for her someone who would not reject or shame her for her body or her passionate ways of expressing herself. He encouraged her to accept him as a "parent" with whom she could express her affections without fear of rejection or shame. Thompson, found this type of "play" therapy central to Ferenczi's relaxation method (Thompson, 1964). His technique was to bring about a "therapeutic regression" or reliving of the trauma to resolve it. By accepting Thompson's kisses, he introduces tenderness and clinical empathy into the analytic encounter. He notes that she has had to forego being "feminine" because it offended her mother. The consequences of this observation have not been fully discussed, though he does allude to her bisexuality and her feminism.

As Ferenczi points out in the *Diary*, his method of acceptance was not always successful; sometimes, it came with unintended consequences. Patients took advantage of his passivity, and he had to take control and bring them back to reality (Dupont, 1988). This in part is why Thompson came to disagree with his method of regression in the service of healing trauma. She did not underestimate the level of aggression a patient might unleash as she wrote later in her essay, "Ferenczi's Relaxation Method" (Thompson, 1964).

Green (1964) commented that her personality was a mix of intense warmth and "a kind of detachment." He tells us, she could manage "to communicate a warm sense of humor and an affectionate smile" despite her practical demeanor (p. 348). Thompson was a classic New Englander— warm, friendly, practical, realistic, private, and understated. This set of cultural characteristics may be misinterpreted as clinical symptoms. In the end, the mixing of patients specifically Severn and Thompson leave room for doubt as to whether Thompson was sexually abused by her father.[14][15]

As Dupont explains:

> What I can say about Ferenczi's intentions is pure hypothesis. It could be a possible explanation of the facts. As the Diary was written at the same time as he did the clinical work with the two women, it could only be a voluntary mixing. But I cannot guarantee the exactness of my explanation.
>
> (Dupont, personal communication, April 15, 2019)

The Importance of the Clinical Diary

The preservation and publication of the *Clinical Diary of Sándor Ferenczi* is an invaluable accomplishment and contribution to the history of psychoanalysis. Judith Dupont deserves not only the credit for this feat, but our appreciation as do the translators, Michael Balint and Nicola Zarday Jackson. They viewed Ferenczi's clinical observations about his patients, himself, and the process of psychoanalytic work as significant to preserve—their persistence over decades to bring this work to fruition is commendable.

Ferenczi's diary, provides a view into Thompson's struggle to express her affection. In her early life and prior to her analysis, she had hidden her feelings leading to an emotional detachment, social isolation, and loneliness. She benefited from Ferenczi's therapeutic techniques—his active approach—including his realness, his therapeutic love, his willingness to extend himself. We know that Thompson learned these clinical innovations firsthand and that she integrated them into her own psychoanalytic practice, making it an interpersonal therapeutic approach.

Key Contributions

The collaborative work of Clara Thompson and Sándor Ferenczi has gone missing in recanting the historical development of Interpersonal Psychoanalysis. The relationship between Thompson and Ferenczi was substantial in personal terms as well as in clinical innovations. As Prince (2018) points out, "The importance of personal and social relations on the development of the interpersonal school . . . "should not be underestimated" (p. 209). Ferenczi's work with Thompson and his other patients led to theoretical and clinical innovations. These innovations were part of Thompson's quest for psychic freedom, but they also became part of her brand of American psychoanalysis. As Benjamin Wolstein said of his analysis with Thompson,

"She took me on a trip, and I took her on a trip. It was a quest for psychic freedom . . . in that context, anything went" (Hirsch, 2000, p. 187). The same was most likely true of Thompson's analysis with Ferenczi.

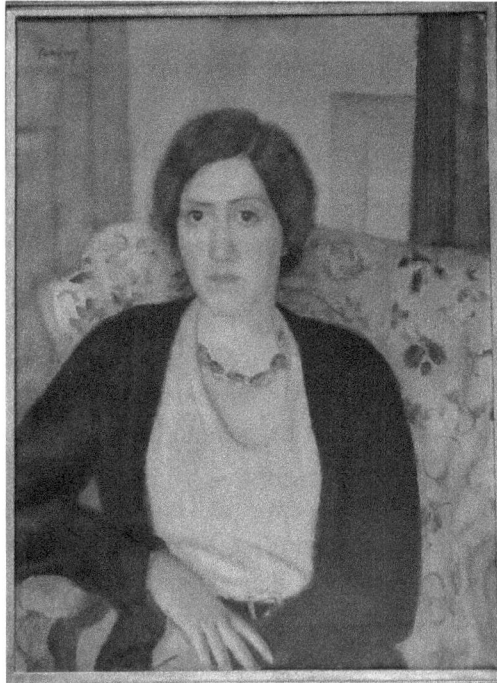

Figure 4.1 Painting of Clara Thompson when she was in her late 20s or early 30s. Original artist unknown. Reprinted with permission, © William Alanson White Institute.

Notes

1 See GG Archives: The future of our past: Social and Cultural History (www
.gjenvick.com/OceanTravel/Brochures/RSL-1926-SecondClassRates.html.)
2 Childhood victimization was, and still is, alarmingly prevalent (Finkelhor,
1997). Data gathered from different countries confirmed the prevalence of
abuse, and that the incidence of childhood sexual abuse, rape, and violence far
exceeds the scope of the problem inferred from officially reported cases . . .
Investigators concluded that "given its 'magnitude' . . . virtually any mental
health professional is going to be dealing with many individuals who have been
sexually abused whether disclosed or not" (p. 101). It is not surprising that Ferenczi's patients frequently reported childhood sexual trauma, what is surprising
is that he took them seriously. See Rachman, A. W. & Klett, S. (2018) Analysis
of the incest trauma: Retrieval, recovery, renewal. Routledge. New York.
3 Rudnytsky (2015) points to how "Freud alleged that Ferenczi had fallen victim to 'mental degeneration' that was manifested in his 'technical innovations'" (p. 140). Later, as noted above, Jones (1957) questioned Ferenczi's
mental health, claiming he was psychotic. Yet, Ferenczi's patient Izette de
Forest astutely suggested—if Ferenczi were really *non compos mentis*, why
would Freud have continued to court him for the job as president of the International? Ferenczi's technical innovations remained hidden or suspect for
decades until the publication of the Freud and Ferenczi correspondence and
the *Clinical Diary*, edited by Judith Dupont (1988).
4 Ferenczi's notes were written over ten months while working with eight
patients. While some were handwritten on scraps of paper and backs of enve-
lopes, eighty percent were on typewritten pages. During the Second World
War, they were kept safe by Ferenczi's wife, Gizella, and then handed off to
Ferenczi's analysand, Michael Balint, who kept them secret for decades. They
cover what Balint (1968) called Ferenczi's "grand experiment," referring specifically to his mutual analysis with Elizabeth Severn in the clinical treatment
of trauma. Judith Dupont, a family friend and prominent psychoanalyst, edited
the final manuscript. Michael Balint and Nicola Zarday Jackson translated it
and made many decisions regarding the text before publication.
5 The editor, Judith Dupont, notes that "sometimes he used several different
abbreviations in referring to one patient." Dupont maintained, "their [patient's]
initials have been altered here according to Ferenczi's own style in the *Diary*."
6 Christopher Fortune (1993) discovered that R.N., in the *Clinical Dairy* was
Elizabeth Severn. William Brennan (2015) successfully identified the remaining patients: Ett. is Izette de Forest; B. is Alice Lowell; O.S. is Natalie Rogers;
N.D./N.H.D. is Roberta (Robbie) Nederhoed; S.I. is Countess Harriot Sigray;
U. is Theodore (Teddy) Miller; and Mrs. G is Anjelika Bijur Frink.
7 Dear Dr. Dupont:

>In conducting a close reading of the Clinical Diary of Sándor Ferenczi, we
>have come to a question that haunts our reading of the material. We wonder
>if the question that worries us has puzzled you in your editing of the Diary.
>In short, could Clara Thompson (Dm.) and Elizabeth Severn (R.N.) have
>been confused in the clinical notes of their analyses?
>   Let me explain how we come to this question. I, Ann D'Ercole, am writ-
>ing a biography of Clara Thompson. I have found in searching the material

on Thompson no evidence in any of Thompson's clinical writings, letters to friends and colleagues or interviews that can verify her father sexually abused her. But there is ample evidence that Elizabeth Severn did suffer sexual abuse by her father.

On the first pages of the Clinical Diary, Ferenczi talks about Dm. in one paragraph and then what seems to be R.N. in the same paragraph as if the two women have been blurred into one. We refer you to the bottom of page two and the top of page three of the Diary.

Ferenczi begins speaking about Dm. "a lady who, 'complying' with my passivity, had allowed herself to take more and more liberties, and occasionally even kissed me." This statement can be verified in various documents including the interview Thompson gave to Eissler in the Freud archives (1952) and with references she makes in her own clinical essays.

It is on page three where Ferenczi says,

As a child, Dm. had been grossly abused sexually by her father, who was out of control; later, obviously because of the father's bad conscience and social anxiety, he reviled her, so to speak. The daughter had to take revenge on her father indirectly, by failing in her own life.

For example, the statement conflicts with data from Green's (1964) biographical essay of Thompson where he reported that Thompson "adored her father" and how he was a "highly successful, self-made man who, beginning as a salesman, had worked himself up to the presidency of one of the outstanding drug companies in the United States" (p. 349). Further, Thompson's mother thought Clara was "her father's favorite" (p. 349). [While not included in the initial letter, it does not mean in any way that having those qualities absolved Thompson's father from being abusive.] Data exists that describes the acrimonious relationship Thompson had with her mother, and she does state that her father never admitted his wrongdoing nor did Adolf Meyer (her teacher).

On the other hand, it is clear that "Elizabeth Severn's father tried to poison her; he sexually abused her; he threw her out of the house; and he cursed her and damned her" (Rachman, 2017, p. 89). In fact, Rachman's research concludes that Severn's father was thought to be a "criminal type who was involved in anti-social behavior." When Ferenczi writes that "The daughter had to take revenge on her father indirectly, by failing in her own life." This too could be Severn not Thompson.

Severn did fail in her life before meeting Ferenczi, whereas Thompson had graduated from medical school and was already a leading figure in the psychoanalytic movement in the United States. Clearly not failing in her life.

To our ears, this sounds like Elizabeth Severn not Thompson who was "grossly sexually abused by her father who was out of control."

Have you ever felt that Ferenczi could have confused the clinical material about Thompson with R.N.?

We greatly appreciate your clarifying whether you have felt this confusion.

Respectfully, Ann D'Ercole and Arnold Rachman

8 Three footnotes added by the editor, Judith Dupont, explain Georg Walter Groddeck was Ferenczi's friend and physician, and Clara Mabel Thompson was Ferenczi's patient between 1928 and 1933. The third footnote refers to the exchange of letters between Freud and Ferenczi in December 1931.

9 Thompson's interview with Eissler helps us understand from her perspective her experience of the so-called "kissing episode":

> "I unfortunately am in a way involved in the struggle with Freud because I was talking with Edith Jackson about his new technique, and she said, "You mean that you actually kiss Ferenczi?" And I said, "Sure, I kiss him any time I want to," And she of course at once went back and told this to Freud and Freud became very upset about this and wrote him quite a letter about it. I must say that Ferenczi was very decent to me. He was very upset naturally, and you see I had proceeded on the theory well if this is what we do, why don't we admit it? and he finally admitted that I was right, that if he was going to do such things, he should admit them and not try to hide it from Freud.
>
> (Freud Thompson-Eissler interview, 1952)

10 In 1943, Thompson stated her agreement with Ferenczi saying clearly, "I agree with him that one of the important factors in producing neurosis is love deprivation in early childhood. Just as the infallible analyst tends to reinforce the patient's attitude towards authority, so the distant mirror-like analyst repeats the love rejection pattern" (p. 64). Rachman (1997) suggests that "Ferenczi used his own traumatic childhood as a gift to his patients by developing his personal empathy into clinical empathy" (p. 214). Brennan (2015) submits that Ferenczi was "enacting his own desire to be the loving mother he never had" (p. 84).

11 The disclosure that she was abused sexually by her father is questionable. It is not consistent with other material in the *Clinical Diary* and it appears mixed with the data from other patients, particularly Elizabeth Severn. Thompson never indicates that she was abused sexually. Green, her friend and analysand, disputed that Dm. was Thompson (see Rachman, 1997, p. 374).

12 Some of his associations seem a forerunner to the work of Julia Kristeva on the concept of the abject. I could find no direct connection between Julia Kristeva and Ferenczi, though Kristeva was in analysis with Ilse Barande, who authored a book on Sándor Ferenczi as well as several articles.

13 In contrast, another patient of Ferenczi's, de Forest (1942) describes what was most important in his trauma theory was not only recalling the memory of early trauma but the reliving of the trauma safely with the analyst (p. 9). Perhaps they both felt Ferenczi's attunement to the subjective experience of the patient: "instilling an atmosphere of openness, safety, and trust, allowing for the free expression of needs, as well as feelings, toward the analyst" (Rachman & Klett, 2018, p. 173) was of utmost importance.

14 Shapiro maintains that even if Thompson was not sexually abused, as Ferenczi's patient, she was in a unique position to bring back his ideas about the reality of abuse and its sequelae. That is true. But Thompson focused her attention elsewhere and prioritized the relationship between the analyst and the patient. Her confusion over whether the "Confusion of Tongues" paper was published is strange. Thompson read the paper; she had stated that the paper was something Ferenczi was working on when she was in treatment

with him and that he read it to Freud, who told him not to present it. The paper is a landmark paper that acknowledges the reality of sexual trauma and the need for empathy and other active clinical techniques. Given its importance, the criticism leveled at Clara Thompson for not prioritizing this message seems warranted. As archaeologists of history, we can only offer our opinions of the data at hand.

15 There are two occasions where Thompson made questionable statements about trauma and abuse. Shapiro (1993) suggests these statements might be indicative of those made by an abuse victim who denies the full extent of "a victim's" helplessness and an overvaluation of their "contributions" (p. 162). The full context of Thompson's (1959) statements shed light on her remarks. She says,

> when a man or woman consults a psychiatrist about marriage difficulties, attention much first be paid to how each is contributing to the situation. There is no such thing as an innocent victim of interpersonal difficulties, except in the case of a very young child.
>
> (p. 239)

Thompson is making the point that a choice of a partner is usually determined by character patterns: "The aggressive person attracts submissive people the masochist attracts those who will make him suffer, the "sucker" is fascinated by the exploiter, etc." (p. 239).

Her statement about rape comes as she asks the question:

> How has it become socially acceptable for a man to insist on his sexual rights whenever he desires? Is this because rape is a possibility, and the woman is physically relatively defenseless? This must have had some influence in the course of society's development. However, it has often been proved that even rape is not easy without some cooperation from the woman. The neurotic condition of vaginismus illustrates that in some conditions even unconscious unwillingness on the part of the woman may effectively block male performance . . . So while the superior physical power of the male may be an important factor . . . other factors are not of a biologic nature, for the participation in sexual relations without accompanying excitement is most obviously possible in human females, although not definitely impossible in other animals.
>
> (Thompson, 1950c, p. 351)

Here Thompson is leading to her culturalist argument that these assumptions are based on a devaluation of the female sex organs.

References

Balint, M. (1968). *The basic fault: Therapeutic aspects of regression*. Tavistock.
Beebe, B., & Lachmann, F. M. (2002). *Infant research and adult treatment: Co-constructing interaction*. The Analytic Press.
Bonomi, C. (1999). Flight into sanity. Jones's allegation of Ferenczi's mental deterioration reconsidered. *International Journal of Psychoanalysis, 80*(3), 507–542.

Brabant, E. (Ed.). (1993). *The correspondence of Sigmund Freud and Sándor Ferenczi: 1920–1933*. Harvard University Press.

Brennan, B. W. (2015). Out of the archive/Unto the couch: Clara Thompson's analysis with Ferenczi. In A. Harris & S. Kuchuck (Eds.), *The legacy of Sándor Ferenczi: From ghost to ancestor* (pp. 77–95). Routledge.

Dupont, J. (Ed.). (1988). *The clinical diary of Sándor Ferenczi* (M. Balint & N. Z. Jackson, Trans.). Harvard University Press.

Dupont, J. (1995). The story of a transgression. *Journal of American Psychoanalytic Association, 43*, 823–834.

Ferenczi, S. (1949a). Confusion of tongues between adults and the child (The language of tenderness and of passion). *International Journal of Psychoanalysis, 30*, 225–230.

Ferenczi, S. (1949b). Notes and fragments (1930–1932). *International Journal of Psychoanalysis, 30*, 231–242.

Finkelhor, D. (1997). Child sexual abuse, challenges facing child protection and mental health professionals. In E. Ullmann & W. Hilweg (Eds.), *Childhood and trauma: Separation, abuse, war* (M. H. Margreiter & K. Henschel trans.) (pp. 101–116). Routledge.

Fortune, C. (1993). The case of "RN": Sándor Ferenczi's radical experiment in psychoanalysis. *Sándor Ferenczi*. News. ALSF No. 2.

Fromm, E. (1964). Foreword. In M. R. Green (Ed.), *Interpersonal psychoanalysis: The selected papers of Clara M. Thompson*. Basic Books.

Green, M. (1964). Her life. In M. R. Green (Ed.), *Interpersonal psychoanalysis: The selected papers of Clara M. Thompson*. Basic Books.

Hirsch, I. (2000). Interview with Benjamin Wolstein. *Contemporary Psychoanalysis, 36*: 187–232.

Jones, E. (1957). *The life and work of Sigmund Freud, Vol. 3: The last phase 1919–1939*. Basic Books.

Perry, H. S. (1982). *Psychiatrist of America: The life of Harry Stack Sullivan*. Belknap Press.

Prince, R. (2018) The influence of Ferenczi on Interpersonal Psychoanalysis in A. Dimitrijevic, G. Cassullo & J. Frankel (Eds.), Ferenczi's influence on contemporary psychoanalytic traditions. (pp. 206–212). Routledge. London and New York.

Rachman, A. W. (1997). *Sándor Ferenczi: The psychotherapist of tenderness and passion*. Jason Aronson.

Rachman, A. W. (2007). Sándor Ferenczi's contributions to the evolution of psychoanalysis. *Psychoanalytic Psychology, 24*(1), 74.

Rachman, A. W. (2012, June 3). *The confusion of tongues between Sándor Ferenczi and Elizabeth Severn*. In Plenary Presentation, The International Sándor Ferenczi Conference, "Faces of Trauma". Budapest, Hungary, Saturday.

Rachman, A. W. (2017). *Elizabeth Severn: The "evil genius" of psychoanalysis*. New York and London: Routledge.

Rachman, A. W. (2021). *Psychoanalysis and society's neglect of the sexual abuse of children, youth and adults: Re-addressing Freud's original theory of sexual abuse and trauma.* New York: Routledge.

Rachman, A. W., & Klett, S. (2018). *Analysis of the incest trauma: Retrieval, recovery, renewal.* New York and London: Routledge.

Roazen, P. (1975). *Freud and his followers.* Da Capo Press.

Rudnytsky, P. L. (2015). The other side of the story: Severn on Ferenczi and mutual analysis. In A. Harris & S. Kuchuck (Eds.), *The legacy of Sándor Ferenczi: From ghost to ancestor* (pp. 134–149). Routledge.

Schachtel, Z. (2016, December 1). (personal communication) interview.

Shapiro, S. A. (1993). Clara Thompson: Ferenczi's messenger with half a message. In L. Aron & A. Harris (Eds.), *The legacy of Sándor Ferenczi* (pp. 159–174). The Analytic Press.

Thompson, C. (1926, January 11). [Letter to Adolf Meyer]. Adolf Meyer Collection 1890–1940; Series I, Unit I/3805, Folder 1. The Henry Phipps Psychiatric Clinic and Baltimore, MD. Alan Mason Chesney Medical Archives of the Johns Hopkins Medical Institutions, Baltimore MD.

Thompson, C. (1931) "Dutiful Child": Resistance. Psychoanalytic Review, 18:426–433.

Thompson, C. (1938). Notes on the psychoanalytic significance of the choice of analyst. *Psychiatry, 1*(2), 205–216.

Thompson, C. (1943). "The therapeutic technique of Sándor Ferenczi": A comment. *International Journal of Psychoanalysis, 24*, 64–66.

Thompson, C. (1944). Ferenczi's contribution to psychoanalysis. *Psychiatry, 7*(3), 245–252.

Thompson, C. (1950a). *Psychoanalysis evolution and development.* Hermitage House.

Thompson, C. (1950b) Introduction in S. Ferenczi, Contributions to psychoanalysis (changed to Sex in psychoanalysis). (no page number) Basic Books, New York.

Thompson, C. (1950c). Some effects of the derogatory attitude towards female sexuality. *Psychiatry, 13*(3), 349–354.

Thompson, C. (1955). Introduction. In M. Balint (Ed.), *Final contributions to the problems and methods of psychoanalysis: The selected papers of Sándor Ferenczi, M.D.* (Vol. 3, pp. 3–4). Basic Books.

Thompson, C. (1964). Ferenczi's relaxation method. In M. R. Green (Ed.), *Interpersonal psychoanalysis: The selected papers of Clara M. Thompson* (pp. 67–71). Basic Books.

Thompson, C. (1988). Sándor Ferenczi, 1873–1933. *Contemporary Psychoanalysis, 24*(2), 182–195.

Chapter 5

The Budapest Years

A Laboratory for a New Psychoanalysis

The City of Budapest

The beautiful city of Budapest had a thriving intellectual life in the early 20th century (Keve, 2018). Its history prior to World War I is complex. In 1867, it had been the co-capital with Vienna of the Dual Monarchy, governing the Hungarian portion of the Austro-Hungarian territory. In *Budapest 1900: A Historical Portrait of a City and Its Culture* (1988), the Hungarian-born historian John Lukacs describes a post-war Budapest that still had important beautiful museums and cultural institutions:

> [B]ut it looks like an empty ballroom. Hungary lost ⅔ of its territory and people by the war, and is barely able to exist. There are traffic cops, every street corner, magnificently turned out in trench coats and swords, but there is no traffic to regulate.
>
> (p. 214)

In the immediate aftermath of the war, a Soviet republic was established in Hungary. It collapsed after a few months and was replaced by a right wing government that stayed in power until 1944. The Jewish population was blamed for attacks against the communists and those who supported them. It was in this anti-Semitic climate that Ferenczi lost his professorship at the University of Budapest and was dismissed from the Budapest Medical Association. Keve (2018) writes:

> Ferenczi had no future in academia, but his work did not require him to be attached to a university. During the 1920s he was kept busy with

DOI: 10.4324/9781003261797-6

his private patients and was prolific in his published work. He considered emigrating, but did not actually take the step. Instead, he travelled to Germany, Austria, the United States, and elsewhere as one of the major figures of the international psychoanalytic community. It was not until 1928 that he held public lectures in Budapest again . . . an easy prosperity returned to Budapest. Jews in trade and the professions were not molested and as the economy improved, they thrived . . . middle class prospered; the cafes were overflowing, intellectual life flourished . . . Sunday afternoon tea dances were frequented by the bourgeoisie . . .

(pp. 16–17)

Budapest was a city of contradictions in this period. According to Lukacs (1988), as time went on, people

breathed freer . . . The air had become lighter. Here and there the city began to sparkle anew. These are not mere figures of speech. They suggest developments on many different levels . . . Financial stability and a measure of industrial prosperity returned. The high standards of education and of publishing climbed to their earlier, prewar standards, even surpassing them in some instances. The years 1921 to 1935 could be (and sometimes are) called the Silver Age of modern Hungarian letters. In the late twenties there was a kind of silvery elegance in the theaters and the drawing rooms and in the appearance of fashionable women in the streets, hotel halls, shops and foyers of Budapest, with a dash of panache that evoked the attention and admiration of foreign visitors . . . tourism had become an important element in the life of the city, especially in the summers. After about 1926 Budapest began to attract tens of thousands of foreign visitors.

(p. 213-214)

Budapest was a trendy destination. Many artists and writers were drawn there, including "Toscanini, Caruso, Horowitz, etc. etc." (p. 214).

By August 1931, when Thompson arrived for her long stay in Budapest, the political climate in Hungary had become tumultuous as the country descended into economic depression. With the rise of Hitler to power in

Germany, Hungary's rulers were soon to align with the fascist Rome to Berlin Axis.

There are no references to these political affairs by Thompson. This may reflect the navel-gazing attitude for which psychoanalysis has been criticized. During her interview with Eissler, Thompson does mention the explosion that caused the train the Vienna Express to plunge into a ravine (see Chapter 1). In the Eissler interview, she mentions Ferenczi's growing concern and his desire to find an island of shelter from what he felt was an approaching storm and her sense of having protection as an American. Beyond that, Thompson makes little reference to political events in Budapest. Perhaps since she could not read Hungarian newspapers or those in German, she was kept somewhat in the dark.

Thompson's Life in Budapest

It was the other, more benign Budapest that Thompson knew. An informative view of her social life in Budapest comes from her Hungarian friend, Dr. Ilona Vass. Vass met Thompson during the summer of 1928. Her essay, published in the *William Alanson White Institute Newsletter* in March 1959, opens a window into Thompson's life there:

Hungary was at the peak of its prosperity at this time and Budapest reflected it. It was a lively, glowing city at the heights of its cultural glory, eager and happy to greet its guests from all over the world. No wonder that it was love at first sight between Clara and the Hungarian capital. She found a charming home in Buda, the ancient part of the city, complete with a cook, Marishka, and a light grey alley cat, Megedge (one more) and soon came to love everything surrounding her. The balmy springs, the hot dry summers, the friendly little restaurants in Buda with their tasty food and gypsy music, the taxi drivers who tried to teach her how to speak Hungarian on her rides there, the tug boats on the Danube, the artesian swimming pools, the lights that transformed the city into a fairyland at night, and the snowy winters in her snugly heated apartment. It was the atmosphere in which her zest for life, her healthy curiosity for experience, and her hunger for knowledge, all found satisfaction and outlet. On her fourth trip she settled down to work with her patients who had traveled from Baltimore to Budapest, to continue their analysis with her. Some of those patients had funds to support their analysis; others did not. The value of Hungarian currency was low, travel was incredibly cheap. Nevertheless, their courage and ingenuity aroused my deepest admiration. During her stay in Budapest Clara never had less than seven patients and for a while she had nine. That means she worked quite a lot since she was seeing her patients multiple times a week. Her sessions with Ferenczi were daily. She often spoke of her enthusiasm for his new approach to analysis, his warmth, and his intuitive humanity.

(p. 2)

Interconnections

During Thompson's stay in Europe, she had many overlapping interpersonal connections. These relationships extended from Vienna to Budapest and, in some ways, echoed today's analytic training institutes; e.g., training analysts conducting multiple analyses and the supervision of candidates, with everyone mixed in classes together, sharing analysts and supervisors. It is a constellation of mostly positive, creatively energizing, and interpersonally complicated relationships. However, the Vienna and Budapest experience was different than that of today as the field was still in its infancy. Professional boundaries were less defined and understood. In some ways, Thompson's time in Budapest was akin to living in a psychoanalytic research laboratory without confidentiality being protected. Despite the imperfections, it is in Budapest where Thompson developed her analytic voice and where she experienced a new psychoanalysis she would bring back to America.

Ernst Falzeder (2019) makes the point that the borders between professional training and personal relationships in psychoanalysis are less defined than its advocates suggest: "Through the personal analysis of the analyst-to-be, each psychoanalyst becomes part of a genealogy, of a family tree, that ultimately goes back to Sigmund Freud and the early pioneers of psychoanalysis" (p. 51). Connecting each psychoanalyst with their mentors—analysts, supervisors, teachers—is illuminating. Clara Thompson's (Hopkins, c. 1920) branch of the family tree begins in Budapest with Ferenczi's and includes his other analysands, Izette de Forest, Alice Lowell (Tufts, c. 1941), and Elizabeth Severn, all early psychoanalytic pioneers. Another branch of this family tree holds friends of Thompson's from medical school in Vienna Edith Jackson (Hopkins, c. 1921) in treatment with Sigmund Freud, and Lucile Dooley (Hopkins, c. 1922) in therapy with Ruth Mack Brunswick (Tufts, c. 1922). By illuminating these "interconnections of psychoanalysts across time and country," the filiations that had previously obscured these early women pioneers have been located in their appropriate time and place (p. 215). This enables both historians to tell a more accurate story and clinical practitioners to see how theories and practices were passed down through the years, thus identifying the sources of influence.

Interconnecting Relationships, Analytic Siblings, Multiple Triangles

Descriptions of Clara Thompson's life in Budapest can seem like a romantic drama series featuring four young women living in the city. There were blurred professional and personal boundaries, romantic relationships, and exchanges of confidences. One can imagine Clara Thompson, Izette de Forest, Alice Lowell, and Elizabeth Severn, all patients of Sándor Ferenczi, gathering together, exchanging ideas, and sharing intimacies as well as harboring jealousies and competitions. As foreigners in a new country their senses of smell and taste and sensitivity to changes in weather heightened the intensity of their experience. They may have sought out each other to feel a sense of home as Americans abroad. Berman (2015) offers a perspective on Thompson's life in Budapest. He asks why

> [Ferenczi] never considered the option of referring new patients, who are intensely involved with an analysand already working with him, to another colleague. Possibly he enjoyed the experience of omniscience enhanced by having multiple sources of information about one's patient, without taking into account the emotional price.

(p. 31)

He seems to single out Ferenczi as if Freud like Ferenczi did not have similar professional and personal relationships (see Roazen, 1975). The ethics and management of clinical boundaries in therapeutic relationships were more fully elaborated much later in the development of the field. Still, boundaries are not as rigid as Berman suggests. Ferenczi's empathic method encouraged the freer expression of feelings and behaviors for both patient and analyst. Ferenczi did express concern about the unintended consequences of his relaxation method (see pgs. 2–3 of the *Clinical Diary*).

Thompson's time in Budapest is interwoven with references to Ferenczi's clinical experimentation and developments. His attempt at mutual analysis was a creative treatment technique he hoped would be helpful to his patients. It was both a groundbreaking advancement in clinical work and conceivably a source of unexamined conflicts. While Freud located the person's internal life as the subject of inquiry in psychoanalytic treatment, Ferenczi saw the inter-subjective as more of a "meeting of minds," to use Lew Aron's (2013) term, a dynamic that occurs in the process of a psychoanalytic encounter. The mutual sharing of subjective experience as a therapeutic technique has become part of the routine practice of interpersonal/relational psychoanalysis that began as Ferenczi's experiment with his patients that included Clara Thompson.

> The secrets of other patients must be divulged by the analyst to the analyzing analysand . . . the patients do not know that I, the analyst, am having myself analyzed (and this by other patient) . . . this "polyg-amous" analysis which roughly corresponds to the group analysis of American colleagues (even if it is not carried out in groups), provides a certain reciprocal control over the various analyses . . . I can report on three analyses that run into one another in connection with me.
>
> (Dupont, 1988, p. 34)

Berman (2015) faults Ferenczi suggesting that he was treating his practice as a group therapy without the actual group process. He wonders if this "virtual group" model of treatment may have "sabotaged Ferenczi's clinical work during this important and fascinating period" (p. 30). However, the success of Ferenczi's work is attested to by Thompson, de Forest, and Severn. Rachman & Klett (2018) also confirm the success of Ferenczi's "trauma analysis."

The people involved in these overlapping relationships that filled Thompson's life in Budapest deserve fuller attention.

Theodore Miller

At the age of 31, Clara Thompson began a relationship with Theodore "Teddy" Miller. On his travel papers, Miller listed Thompson's address at the Hotel Bellevue in Budapest as his own and Thompson as his closest relative, suggesting the intimacy of their connection. Miller, patient U. in Ferenczi's *Diary*, is described as a handsome and quirky businessman. A historical search of Theodore Miller or Ancestry.com shows his WWII draft card which indicates he worked for the Miller Rockwool Company, a manufacturer of insulation, an advancement that allowed buildings to hold heat and keep out dampness. The draft card also confirms that he had a scar on his face (see Brennan, 2018). Upon his return to the states, Miller lived for a time with Helen Ney in Detroit in the 1940s. The trail of his whereabouts falls off after that.

We know Theodore Miller was born in Poland in 1902 and came to the United States in 1914. Brennan (2018) describes him as an untrustworthy businessman and known "philanderer" (p. 88). By 1931, he was in Budapest, where he met Clara Thompson. They seem to have been together from 1931 to 1933 and returned to New York together on July 4, 1933, following Ferenczi's death.

The letter from Thompson to Voss demonstrates the ambivalence of their relationship: "I clung to Teddie and he to me but gradually it became apparent that one of us must get free because we were in a way holding each other down" (Shapiro, 1993, p. 168).

The *Diary* provides a glimpse into his interpersonal struggles. Thompson and Miller's relationship is referred to in a passage in the *Diary* where Ferenczi describes how U. (Teddy Miller) had fallen in love with an "elderly lady" presumably Dm. (Thompson was nine years his senior). In the *Diary*, Ferenczi notes that Miller "complained about her but could not do without her." Ferenczi writes:

> he is carrying on affairs with five or six other women and makes no secret of this information from the lady {Thompson}. The lady takes his courtship seriously and begins to behave as though she were the fiancée of the young man, a step that the patient does not oppose strongly enough. At the same time sexual relations with her are more satisfying, on occasion, than with any of the others. Finally, he exposes her to the danger of infection. This leads to moments of manifest anger and hatred

on the part of the woman. Although this affected U. painfully, he still had friendly feelings toward her afterward. Soon after this, however, the woman began to try to regain his love, as though she had forgiven him; she showed herself hurt and depressed, as it were, by his behavior. At a sudden reversal of feelings in U. again; if he was previously somewhat sad about the inevitable separation and happy to have genuine feelings, even gratitude and friendship, now he feels tied down once more (obligation) and compelled to help her and stay with her. At the same time, jealousy toward another young man flares up again.

(Dupont, 1988, p. 207)

From Ferenczi's perspective, Teddy's feelings for Thompson were ambivalent at best. He thoughtlessly exposed her to a sexually transmitted disease and she responded with rage. Yet, Thompson felt sorry for him and wanted Ferenczi to help her out get away from Miller's clinging dependency. Earlier in the *Diary*, Ferenczi writes: "Dm. demands from me . . . that I should become a good mother to U . . . I must admit that I love U. (Daddy!) just as much as I love her" (p. 125). There is a gender fluidity involved with Ferenczi becoming a "good mother" while he plays the role of "Daddy." Ferenczi did not like Miller, so loving him the way Thompson was asking was very difficult. Berman (2015) speculates that Ferenczi "felt dismayed about Teddy's attitude toward women (including Thompson), his multiple simultaneous affairs, and risking his lovers' health because he was infected with gonorrhea by a prostitute" (p. 32).

Ferenczi felt Thompson (Dm.) was using Miller (U.) as a defensive wedge against the analysis by as he claimed, "shifting her love and interest to a young man . . ." Thompson suggests she will sacrifice her interest in Miller for the analysis (Dupont, 1988, p. 57), Berman (2015) posits:

the triangle created between Clara, Teddy and Sándor must have been quite tense and conflictual for all three; it was expressed in two separate analyses, in which the needs of the patients might have been irreconcilable; and it may have made it doubly difficult for Ferenczi to work through his complex countertransference reactions to these two patients. These countertransference feelings may have included jealousy, protectiveness toward Clara who got involved with a destructive man, a wish to disclose to her Teddy's secrets (gonorrhea, other lovers) while being ethically inhibited from doing so, anger toward Teddy for his conduct toward someone personally known to the analyst, and so on.

(p. 32)

One may wonder if there was a reciprocal erotized element in Thompson and Ferenczi's relationship enacted outside of the treatment through Theodore Miller? The same can be asked about Ferenczi and Miller's relationship. What was Thompson's role in the enactment? Thompson had called Ferenczi's relaxation technique "play therapy." Did she borrow the term from Anna Freud's play therapy project? She would have heard the term from her friends Jackson and Dooley who were working with Anna Freud in the development of play therapy. One can imagine the many conversations between these women about their work. Berman (2015) views these triangles as being charged with countertransference feelings including "jealousy, protectiveness toward Clara who got involved with a destructive man, a wish to disclose to her Teddy's secrets (gonorrhea, other lovers) while being ethically inhibited from doing so, anger toward Teddy for his conduct toward someone personally known to the analyst, and so on" (p. 33). Ferenczi also admitted he would have preferred to have a mutual analysis with his patient S. I. (Sigray) rather than Elizabeth Severn since he found S.I. "capable of kindness and selflessness, while in R. N.'s case one always has the feeling that she is constantly pursuing a goal that is finally selfish" (Dupont, 1988, p. 45). These were complicated triangles no doubt excited and confused each of the participants.

Izette de Forest

Izette de Forest is identified as patient Ett. in the *Clinical Diary*. She is a less known collaborator of Ferenczi's who later became a respected psychoanalyst and author of the *Leaven of Love* (1954). Much of what is known about de Forest's life comes from a biographical essay by William B. Brennan (2009) Ferenczi's Forgotten Messenger: The Life and Work of Izette de Forest. That work establishes her place in psychoanalytic history and enriches our understanding of de Forest and her relationship with Thompson and Ferenczi.

According to Brennan (2009), de Forest came from "good New England stock" (p. 432) with a "pioneering spirit" (p. 427). At the age of 16, she became engaged and was immediately sent to Europe by her family with the hope of ending the romance. On her return, she enrolled at Bryn Mawr College. In 1908, she became engaged to Henry Strong Dennison (Denny), the brother of her close friend. He ended the engagement days before she turned twenty-one. Given to the dramatic, de Forest wrote in her diary, "All the light has gone out of the world" (Brennan, 2009, p. 433). Then she met and married Alfred Victor de Forest. Two days after she married Alfred, her previous boyfriend (Dennison) committed suicide. His death had a lasting effect on her.

Her husband, Alfred, was a metallurgist who later became an MIT professor. He was in treatment with Ferenczi for five months. Brennan (2009) reports that de Forest wanted her husband to be "a Ferenczi in magnetics" (p. 433). In fact, Alfred de Forest discovered a technique for detecting cracks in steel by magnetizing it and showering it with carbon particles. It won him the Reed Award of the Institute of Aeronautical Sciences in 1938. Brennan points to "an uncanny parallel" between Ferenczi and Alfred de Forest where Ferenczi is stressing the uncovering of early infantile trauma as cracks in the psychic structure,[1] and Alfred de Forest is detecting hairline cracks and fractures in metal. Ferenczi wrote to him on January 25, 1926:

> It interested me very much that you continue to find resemblances between the ways in which the elements of the inorganic material are connected and the interactions of the elements of the psyche. I always regretted not to know more of the life of the materials, [I mean physics and chemistry] and envy you for the opportunity, to work those interesting inquiries.

(p. 434)

Izette de Forest's interest in psychoanalysis began with her reading of Freud's *The Interpretations of Dreams*. A sexual boundary violation occurred with her first analyst, Frederick Pierce. "As she reported to Alfred in a letter on October 6, 1925, "a powerful erotic transference developed, which Pierce could not refrain from consummating." Brennan tells us that de Forest went into treatment following this event (Brennan, 2009, p. 436).

We learn further that De Forest's husband Alfred was a cousin of Dorothy Tiffany Burlingham, Anna Freud's life companion. The de Forest family socialized with the Burlingham household and with the Freuds.

The de Forests had two children, Taber de Forest, born in 1913, and Judith Brasher de Forest, born in 1915.

According to Brennan (2009) Izette de Forest had a one-year treatment with Ferenczi in Budapest beginning in 1925. He describes how

> Elizabeth Severn had already begun her analysis, and the two American women dined together on several occasions at the Ritz . . . During her year in Budapest, Alfred joined Izette and was himself in analysis with Ferenczi for five months, some of this occurring in Baden, where Izette became acquainted with Georg Groddeck . . .
>
> She continued her treatment with Ferenczi when he came to New York in the fall of 1926 to lecture at the New School for Social Research (Tsuruta, 2005) and through the spring of 1927; then, in keeping with the Hungarian tradition, she started control analysis— that is, supervision—with him at this time. During their visit to the States, Ferenczi, along with his wife, spent weekends at the de Forest home, including over Christmas of 1926.
>
> (p. 437)

Concurrent with Thompson's time in Budapest, de Forest spent

> the summers of 1929–1931 in Europe meeting with Ferenczi. He presented her with a Certificate in the name of the Training Committee of the Hungarian Psychoanalytic Society, dated Budapest, June 1929, which stated that she had completed a personal analysis of fifteen months and control analysis with three patients.
>
> (Brennan, 2009, p. 437)

In her book, *The Leaven of Love* (de Forest, 1954), she pays homage to Ferenczi's ideas, particularly his notions about the curative power of love in the analytic relationship:

> It was my privilege to be in analysis with Sándor Ferenczi in 1925–1927, at the time when he was becoming acutely aware of

his dissatisfaction with some of the crucial aspects of the Freudian approach and of the art of uncovering and restoring the underlying inborn personality . . . My therapeutic analysis and training under his guidance were followed throughout his last years by conversations and discussions on the subject of psychoanalysis . . . in my subsequent professional work I have discovered more deeply the true significance of his theories, and have devoted my psychoanalytic practice to their development.

(pp. xi-xii)

In her analysis with Ferenczi, de Forest had recalled that as a child, her nurse would masturbate her. When she told her mother the nurse was dismissed but de Forest felt "intense shame." (Brennan, 2009, p. 445). Ferenczi's intense re-living techniques had helped her recall this shameful episode.

In her essay "The Therapeutic Technique of Sándor Ferenczi" (1942), de Forest lays out Ferenczi's modifications of Freud's techniques and his implementation of his new methods:

Ferenczi's analytic treatment had no set limits. To help the patient gradually to gain the strength to re-experience the original trauma or traumatic series of experiences was always his hope. Or, if it was a case of long exposure to a cruel environment, as is so frequently true, to re-experience this exposure over and over again, and with increasing tension, seemed essential to a permanent cure . . . His chief part, in addition to the application of his skill in understanding and in interpretation, should consist in raising the tension between himself and the patient in proportion to the patient's endurance. This . . . means taking an active part in a highly emotional relationship. The purpose . . . is to strengthen the patient, but much more importantly to bring finally and very carefully to a head the threatening dramatic crisis . . . In truth, this is a re-birth. The essential characteristics of parenthood, therefore, were to Ferenczi the essential characteristics of the analyst. Clear understanding of oneself, depth of feeling and human kindness, humility, high imagination, great patience and endurance, fearlessness, a capability to learn and an ability to teach by example rather than by precept—these are as necessary elements in the analyst's capacity as is his carefully acquired skill. Sándor Ferenczi little knew, as he so painstakingly and with much opposition laboured at his psycho-analytical research.

(de Forest, 1942, p. 20)

Clara Thompson (1943), in her review of de Forest's work, offered her own take on some of Ferenczi's ideas noting:

> I am a pupil of Ferenczi and for over ten years, I have made use of some of his techniques in my psycho-analytic work. In the course of time I have discarded several of his ideas and confirmed the validity of others. I think that my conclusions, which are somewhat different from Mrs. de Forest's, would be a valuable addition to her paper . . . He sought for ways to make the analysis vivid and living. He believed that the patient is ill because he has not been loved, and that he needs from the analyst the positive experience of acceptance, i.e. love. This could not be given by a mirror. He therefore came to the conviction that the real personality of the analyst plays a part in the therapeutic process, that his blind spots, short-comings and also positive qualities are felt intuitively by the patient, who reacts to them. In consequence, any consideration of the patient's attitudes should include an evaluation of the reality relationship to the analyst, and a therapeutic situation can only exist when the analyst has a positive feeling of acceptance for the patient . . . The difficulty lies in the definition of the word "love." I think Ferenczi was not entirely clear on this matter. His idea was that the analyst must give the patient all the love he needs. The basic need of every child is to be accepted, to feel himself secure with one individual. This type of acceptance is also what the patient needs. I think, however, Ferenczi tended to confuse the idea that the patient must be given all the love he needs with the idea he must be given all the love he demands. Obviously, the two are not identical.

(p. 64)

De Forest and Thompson emphasized different aspects of Ferenczi's work, with de Forest finding placing value in the reliving experience and Thompson focusing on the interplay of analyst's and patient's personalities. Having recovered her original childhood trauma in her work with Ferenczi, de Forest underscored the importance of the living-through of the trauma in the regression and transference. Brennan (2009) describes an undated journal entry possibly from the 1950s, where de Forest mentions "Clara's lack of appreciation for Ferenczi" (p. 451). Brennan speculates that de Forest "sensed some reservation in Thompson's attitude." Perhaps she felt that, in their rivalry, her devotion as a dutiful daughter had prevailed (p. 452).

While Thompson is seen as Ferenczi's major protégée in North America, Brennan (2009) recognizes Izette de Forest as his "forgotten messenger" (p. 247). He argues: the pivotal role played by de Forest in the dissemination of Ferenczi's ideas has been overlooked (p. 429). What has also been overlooked is the passionate relationship between Izette de Forest and Alice Lowell as revealed in the many letters from Lowell to de Forest (courtesy of Henry Taves).

Brennan (2009) surmises that a sibling competitiveness may have spurred Thompson and de Forest to write about Ferenczi. On the other hand, they were supportive of each other and intimate with the details of their inner experience as demonstrated by the frequency of their correspondence. A sign of their trust in one another is that de Forest sent both her children for analysis with Clara Thompson. Her daughter Judy was in treatment with Thompson for over a decade. In her interview with Eissler, Thompson suggests that Judy emerged from their work together a very happy person.

In a letter dated October 7, 1932, Thompson wrote de Forest about her patient's death and her attempt to follow Ferenczi's techniques.

> I've had one tragedy this year. My psychotic patient is having another psychosis. I knew why. Following Ferenczi's method I have tried to find a fault in me and doubtless it is but Ferenczi thinks now that perhaps psychotics need more security than any human being can give them. I know that my being in analysis may have been very hard for her but she was like a baby in reacting to the deep undercurrents in me and I know that she became ill in a very difficult time in my analysis. That is the nearest I can come to my fault.
>
> (Brennan, 2009, p. 447)

In a letter to de Forest dated October 7, 1932, Thompson noted how much she missed the presence of English speakers in Budapest with whom she could share ideas: "I think if I had more competition, I would feel more stimulated to put my ideas in writing" (p. 450). Brennan writes:

When Izette's book was published a decade later, Clara wrote a note of appreciation on April 26, 1954, for having been sent a copy, but took the opportunity to emphasize the differences between them even more starkly:

> I've just finished reading your book and I found it very stimulating, [...] especially the first part with excellent case material. Although you probably know I no longer put as much stress on recovering the early traumatic experience as Ferenczi did[,] I still agree that the powerful emotional experience in the analysis with the "loving" analyst is what produces its cure. I put loving in quotes because I think that both you and I do not spare the stern probing of destructive attitudes which I think Ferenczi tended to overlook. And people do not always think of such approaches as being a part of love, although I am sure they are. I notice you quote from his Wiesbaden paper. Is that in the posthumous publications? I have never run across it. I am sure your book will bring hope to a lot of people and I hope it will help analysts to think more about being human beings.
>
> (pp. 451–452)

Her daughter may have been in treatment with Thompson when she wrote to her on May 9, 1944, following Thompson's presentation of her paper on Ferenczi. De Forest had been the discussant.

> I hope you will see why I talked of "Thalassa" and also why I only enlarged on the reliving part of F's theory. I don't think Clara really grasps what it meant to him because she didn't experience it with him, he was more or less lost in his endeavor to re-create a good childhood. One can only get the whole of his theory by seeing what he was doing from 1926–1933. She happened in at the tail end. He didn't live long enough to synthesize the whole theory into one unit. That remains for us to do.
>
> (Brennan, 2009, p. 451)

De Forest proposes the notion that Thompson missed the whole of what Ferenczi was constructing because she was with him only in chunks during most of those years, in contrast to de Forest, who had a more sustained, consistent relationship with him.

Like Thompson, de Forest undertook an analysis with Erich Fromm following her treatment with Ferenczi (Brennan, 2009).[2] Thompson and de Forest remained close friends throughout their lives.

The topic of bisexuality is frequently discussed within this group of analytic siblings. Following affairs with several men, in 1930 de Forest fell in love with Alice Lowell, whom she encouraged to travel to Budapest and enter treatment with Ferenczi. Lowell was in touch with Ferenczi up until his last days.

De Forest and Ferenczi had similar experiences of sexual abuse as children. Brennan (2009) notes that in de Forest's analysis she

> uncovered that at an earlier age she had had a nurse that would masturbate her. Upon her mother's discovery of this, the nurse was dismissed . . . Izette felt intense shame. She realized that when she experienced rejection and abandonment by men she would turn to women for solace.
>
> (p. 445)

In an extended notation on May 17, 1932, Ferenczi offers a theory that a heterosexual trauma leads to homosexuality in women. He cites patient Ett. (de Forest) as an example, noting:

Heterosexual trauma, flight into (female) homosexuality.

> 1. Patient Ett. returned home at her own wish . . . Relationship to her husband unsatisfactory . . . came to me for control analysis in America. It turned out that she knew all along . . . of an indiscretion, about my sympathy for another woman patient. Perhaps out of revenge . . . she arranged things as follows: she became reconciled with her husband after he confessed his infidelity . . . she fell in love with a married man, who will not divorce his wife . . . she fell in love with a very attractive girl and from then on divided her libido among all of them . . . she revealed her dissatisfaction with me, by developing an intellectual transference for a colleague in America . . . 2. This same girl comes to me for analysis, constantly reiterating her fidelity to her friend, the woman mentioned above. After a frank discussion about my dissatisfaction, her self-confidence suddenly increases . . .

she feels certain that she can, whenever she wants to, seduce any person, male or female . . . she regards herself as a public menace because of her skill in seduction; she gets the impression that I, too, am becoming libidinally dependent on her. The pleasure she takes in herself and the world at large often causes persistent genital sensations, a kind of prolonged orgasm. Fragments from a frequent dream . . . she is lying on the slightly sloping concrete floor of the subway and a mass of slime, in constant danger of sliding between the rails. Her right leg is paralyzed. She hangs on with one finger in a hole; another woman pins her down with her own weight; she is also slipping downward in the same dangerous manner. The patient gets this woman off by sticking the woman's fingers, which have been gripping her convulsively, into the same hole. Finally, however, even so, her own strength gives away and she falls onto the rails, that is, she loses consciousness. Then she sees herself struggling away from the railway track, following a complicated path toward a house, where she is kindly invited in by an elderly gentleman (from the balcony). On the way she feels dreadfully ill, she is aware of a terrible nausea, she falls down, grabs a valuable vase as a receptacle, and vomits continuously like a fountain, finally even on the floor, until everything is awash. The fluid has a strange taste and there are seeds in it. She comes to from the second fit a fainting, as described above. On the way to the place where she vomited, there are people who accuse her unjustly. As she is walking, her right leg becomes twice its size, and she has to walk with flexed knees in order to be able to walk at all.

(Dupont, 1988, pp. 108–109)

Homosexuality and psychoanalysis have had a problematic history. There were misguided efforts to assign a biological, psychological, and environmental etiology to homosexuality working under the hypothesis that there was "normal" and "abnormal" sexual behavior. Drescher (2008) argues that those theories broadly occupied three categories, "normal variation . . . a phenomenon that occurs naturally . . . pathology, treating adult homosexuality as a disease . . . and immaturity, regarding aspects of homosexuality at a young age as a normal step toward adult heterosexuality . . . a phase to be outgrown" (p. 444).

As Drescher (2008) argues, Freud was tolerant for his time, demonstrated by his signed 1930 petition to decriminalize homosexuality. Yet, although he did not consider homosexuality an illness, his theory did not quite constitute a clean bill of health—calling someone immature, rather than sick, is not as offensive, but neither appellation is particularly respectful (p. 446).

In a confusing notation, Ferenczi begins by citing Ett. Later, as if he was not discussing her from the beginning, he refers back to her, noting he left aside the traumatic aspects of the dream and instead, "I focus on her being pinned down by another woman and her extraordinary way of freeing herself . . . Probably this means she not only had to endure the trauma but also had to preserve artistically the tranquil life of her mother by keeping it a secret" (Dupont, 1988, p. 109).

In his second interpretation, he

> points toward mutual masturbation; she trains her mother, with whom she associated herself sexually in a compulsive manner (hence the relationship with Ett.), to gratify herself. It is only when she probes beyond the homosexuality that she arrives at real events, that is, the heterosexual trauma, which left her with an enormous yearning for enormous physical satisfaction. Should the analysis succeed in overcoming her anxiety and shame at this immense eroticism, then she will totally renounce her homosexuality (out of regard for her mother). There remains only one problem: what is to happen in reality to the prematurely awakened libido.
>
> (p. 110)

Ferenczi theorizes:

> female homosexuality is in fact a very normal thing, just as normal as male heterosexuality. Both man and woman have in the beginning the same female love-object (the mother) . . . Fixation on the father or on the male sex, in contrast, is thoroughly abnormal; above all, it is in contradiction with anatomy, which (contrary to Freud) I consider fundamentally determining in psychology . . . the girl's relationship with her mother is much more important than that with her father.
>
> (pp. 78–79)

This quote from Ferenczi is confusing. He tells the reader he is speaking about de Forest but ends with a dream in which he refers back to de Forest as if he was not speaking about her. Could the dream possibly be that of Alice Lowell? The potential mix-up aside, the point here is that he is offering a reparative theory of sexuality.

This extension of Freud's theory suggesting that homosexuality could be changed became damaging for decades (Drescher, 1998). Drescher (2008) describes a comprehensive history of psychoanalytic attitudes toward homosexuality locating them in the political, cultural, and personal contexts where they were formulated. Through the years, analysts have taken positions that either facilitated or obstructed tolerance and acceptance.

Alice Lowell

There were two sets of patients in Ferenczi's practice who were engaged in romantic relationships with one another: Thompson and Miller, and Lowell and de Forest.

Alice Lowell (1906–1982) is patient B. in the *Diary*. She was from Concord, Massachusetts, not far from Thompson's hometown of Providence. She attended the prestigious Milton Academy, traveled to Paris and Switzerland, and studied music. She was in treatment with Ferenczi from 1930 to 1933. In 1941, she earned her medical degree from Tufts Medical School. Her original goal was to become a psychoanalyst. Instead, however, she chose internal medicine as her specialty (Brennan, 2015a). Lowell lived in New York City until 1949 and was on the faculty of Columbia University's College of Physicians and Surgeons. From 1947 to 1951, she was a clinical professor at New York University and in private practice. She returned to New England to the faculty of Boston University's School of Medicine and at Massachusetts Memorial Hospital. She conducted research about blood-volume expanders, in collaboration with her brother, Dr. Francis Cabot Lowell. She also was an expert on asthma, from which she suffered. She was Medical Director and Chief of Medicine at New England Hospital, Boston, MA. In her obituary (*Boston Globe*, 4/23/82), she is described by friends as a woman with great style and a commanding presence but also a warm and caring way with people. She was also an accomplished musician. Alice Lowell was in a long-term relationship with Annella Brown, MD, one of the nation's first board-certified women surgeons.

As Brennan (2009) tells the story, Izette de Forest "fell in love" with Alice Lowell in 1930. She gave Alice a "thin gold Carder band inscribed with their initials as a symbol of their relationship" (p. 443). Soon after Lowell traveled to Budapest to begin treatment with Ferenczi.

Like most of the patients included in the *Clinical Diary*, Alice Lowell experienced sexual trauma:

> In the course of the first session, induced by the "egg dream" complete reproduction of sensations: the smell of alcohol and tobacco as on the breath of her attacker; violent twisting of her hands at the wrists, a feeling of trying to push off with the palms the weight of a gigantic body; then a feeling of pressing weight on her chest, obstruction of her breathing by clothing, suffocations, violent stimulation . . . of her lower extremities; a most painful sensation in the abdomen with a marked rhythm, a feeling of leakage; finally the feeling of dying as though nailed to the floor, bleeding that will not stop, the sight of an evil, peering face. Then only the sight of the enormous legs of a man, arranging his clothes, leaving her to lie there.
>
> (Dupont, 1988, p. 21)

By working to intensify the emotional experience, Lowell recalled the sexual trauma: "Her awareness of sexual trauma first occurred through somatic memory, a characteristic experience for incest survivors" (Rachman, 1997, p. 381).

Lowell was a favorite of Ferenczi's. He gave her a portrait of himself with the inscription:

> To an exceptionally excellent pupil, Alice Lowell (Concord, Mass.) From her teacher and friend. Budapest, 12.iii.1933.
>
> (Brennan, 2009, p. 446)

Brennan (2009) points to another significant reference:

> From a second reference in the *Diary* where Ferenczi discusses homosexual relationships in women, it would appear that Alice is patient B. Moreover, the entry on May 10, 1932 describes how Ferenczi had

made a "psychoanalytic confession" (Dupont, 1988, p. 103) of his never-before-expressed dislike of their homosexual relationship that confirmed what B. had intuited.

(p. 443)

Ferenczi was also aware of the complications of the triangle that included him, Lowell, and de Forest. In a letter (March 1, 1932), he writes that de Forest may be holding back in her correspondence to Alice in order to protect him:

> You surely know that I get notice also of your communication to Alice, too. Please don't go in your loyalty to me too far; you must know that you are not obliged in any respect and have full freedom of action and of speech. It is not you but I who has to carry the possible consequences of my own mistakes, or of actions which you regard as such.
>
> (Brennan, 2009, p. 444)

In Thompson (1941), a young woman whose life may be partly based on Lowell's is depicted. The essay speaks to a woman whose parents prevented her from developing her interests in her desired career:

> A young woman announced her wish to study medicine. Both parents disapproved and persuaded her to seek her career in music. She acceded to their wishes and spent several years in study. At the end of that time, she remained dissatisfied and again expressed her wish to study medicine. This time the parents persuaded her to take up nursing. When she had completed this course, she again asked to be allowed to study medicine and finally obtained her wish. She proved to have outstanding ability.
>
> (p. 3)

Edith Banfield Jackson

Edith Jackson had multiple early losses in her life and later becomes intertwined in a number of overlapping relationships, including her connection to Thompson, Freud, Ferenczi, and Lucile Dooley (see Chapter 3).

Born in Colorado, Jackson was one of six children. In his historical study of Jackson's treatment with Freud, Lynn (2003) describes the death of her sister, aged nine months, a loss from which Jackson's mother never recovered. Four years after her child's death, Jackson's mother fatally shot herself. When Jackson learned that her mother had committed suicide, she was being cared for by a loving aunt, Edith Colby Banfield. Another untimely death marked Jackson's life when her aunt died of an acute illness. Jackson's father brought into the home a "domineering, humorless, and moralistic" caretaker who turned out to be physically abusive to the children (p. 610). The children rebelled, except for Jackson who coped by trying to obey. She later wished she had rebelled like her siblings. Edith went on to attend Vassar then Johns Hopkins School of Medicine. She graduated in 1921, a year after Clara Thompson. In the fall of 1927, before beginning her practice, "she decided to undergo psychoanalysis with Lucille Dooley, hoping to resolve 'persistent depression and low self-esteem'" (p. 611). As Silberman (1998) reports,

> Seven months into that analysis and with no end in sight, Jackson began a residency in psychiatry at St. Elizabeth's Hospital. She was still in analysis and had nearly completed her residency when she received word in October 1929 from an old friend, Dr. Smiley Blanton, that Freud, with whom Blanton was then in analysis, would soon have a free hour for which she might apply.
>
> (p. 95)

She underwent a second analysis, a "training analysis" with Sigmund Freud, in Vienna at the age of 35. Lynn (2003) points out that when Jackson arrived in Vienna in 1930, she learned that Freud was analyzing his daughter, Anna. She did not think this was controversial; "she simply saw it as an illustration of his remarkable abilities" (Roazen, 1995, p. 99) rather than egregious. Freud recommended a room for her to rent, and she began a six-days-a-week analysis that increased in frequency to, at times, eight hours a week. Ten months after beginning her treatment, she wrote to her sister: "One of the reasons I sought analysis was to discover why I, a presumably normally healthy and intelligent girl, was steadily growing old without making the normal heterosexual contacts and experiences" (Lynn, 2003, p. 612). Silberman (1998) found that a year later, Jackson understood her therapeutic task to be "remember[ing] the things in the past whose forgetting has kept me from finding satisfaction anywhere" (p. 96). Freud identified for her the importance of her recalling, accepting, and mourning her mother's suicide.

As noted by Lynn (2003), Freud held strong feelings for Jackson. As a symbol of his affection, he gave her both an antique stone that she had set into a ring and

> a puppy, Fo, a daughter of Yofi, Freud's chow . . . he invited her to Berlin . . . to continue analysis there . . . Freud wrote to Edith Jackson at the close of his summer vacation that he expected good results from her analysis . . . you can imagine that we talk about you at home . . . she met Freud's immediate family during the analysis . . . Freud also told Edith Jackson about his opinions of some of the people around him . . . there were least two instances when Freud gave information to Edith Jackson about his analysand. In a session . . . he described Dorothy Burlingham's dream . . . During her analysis . . . Edith Jackson socialized in a circle of people who were close to Freud and who had been, or were being analyzed by him . . . Irmarita Kellars Putnam [c.1921] was a classmate of Edith Jackson at Johns Hopkins . . . During Irmarita's analysis she and Edith spent a great deal of time together . . . they kept up a fully comprehensive discussion of both of their analyses; Freud knew about his ongoing dialogue, and never objected to it . . . their socializing including with Lucille Dooley.
>
> (p. 615)

Jackson had other complicated relationships, including one with her first analyst, Dooley, who was also Clara Thompson's close friend from medical school. Jackson had a complex relationship with Freud's son Martin, who was married. In a letter to Jackson, he wrote:

> Today a letter came . . . confirming what I knew already from my father: that you had left the idea of coming back to work in Vienna and that you had left me. This is very painful. I feel more lonely now than ever. I am with love and rather hard feeling yours.
>
> (p. 616)

After reviewing the "epistolary and photographic evidence of Jackson's relationship with Martin Freud," Silberman (1998) concluded that Jackson did not have "a sexual affair" with Martin Freud but that "they loved each other" (p. 98). Their story hints at an enactment that implicates Freud and his son as powerfully as it does Jackson and her feelings for Freud.

Edith Jackson's letters to her sister continued to reflect her loneliness following her treatment. In 1936, she expected to return to Vienna but decided to stay in the United States. The details of the termination of her work with Freud are unclear.

When Jackson returned home, she did not practice psychoanalysis; rather, she used her analytic knowledge and training differently. She became a nationally recognized member of hospital-based academic pediatricians, obstetricians, and child psychiatrists.

> The group included Benjamin Spock, Erik Erikson, Ernst Kris . . . who deplored the impersonality, authoritarianism, and rigidity of "modern," "scientific" obstetrics and pediatrics, believed that a patient's psychological well-being was as important as her somatic status, and thus worked to "humanize" both the training of doctors and the practice of medicine in the United States at mid-century . . . as director of the Yale Rooming-In Research Project from 1946 to 1953, Jackson applied her psychoanalytic insights and pioneered so notably in three areas—preventive pediatrics, "family centered" maternity and infant care, and parent-infant "bonding" (decades before that concept became modish)—that both the American Academy of Pediatrics and the American Psychiatric Association gave her their coveted annual awards in the 1960s after her retirement.
>
> (Silberman, 1998, p. 99)

Silberman views Jackson's analysis with Freud as successful, despite what she calls a curious pattern of ups and downs in her medical career. Jackson's work was distinguished and her personal life appears to have been rewarding.

Decades after her analysis with Freud, Edith Jackson wasn't sure if her analysis had helped her though Freud believed it had. She admitted she did feel more relaxed. Viewing Jackson from another perspective, Lynn (2003) describes the blurred boundaries that existed between Jackson and her friends and fellow analysands:

> During her analysis, Edith Jackson socialized in a circle of people who were close to Freud and who had been, or were being, analyzed

by him. She believed that Freud was seeing five analysands regularly, with others on an intermittent basis (Roazen, 1995, p. 102). To some extent, she reached an understanding of how Freud related to these various people. Beginning in the first month, and again for a number of occasions, she went to dinner at Ruth Mack Brunswick's home; she knew Ruth's husband Mark Brunswick and his brother, . . . All three were analysands of Freud.

(p. 616)

This was the model of analytic behavior set by Freud and repeated within Ferenczi's circle. The group of women who were Ferenczi's patients in Budapest replicated this analytic model; they were intertwined in their daily lives. They no doubt dined with each other, shopped together, and took walks around the city, as friends might do. The *Clinical Diary* notes them swimming together at the Gellert pool (Dupont, 1988).

Clara Thompson and Edith Jackson were friends since medical school; they would customarily compare notes on their treatments—as Jackson did with her other medical school friends. It is within this context that Thompson told Jackson she could kiss Papa Ferenczi any time she wanted.

Irmarita Kellars Putnam, Jackson's classmate at Johns Hopkins, was in treatment with Freud. She helped her arrange for Jackson's analysis with him. Lynn (2003) maintains that Putnam and Jackson spent a great deal of time together, and Roazen (1995) points to how "they kept up a fully comprehensive discussion of both of their analyses; Freud knew about this ongoing dialogue, and never objected to it" (p. 99). As we have noted, their socializing included Lucille Dooley, another Johns Hopkins graduate, and Jackson's first analyst. The exchange of information about their analyses was commonplace in the group of Hopkins graduates, as was competition and rivalry. Jackson thought of herself as Freud's favorite. Brennan (2011) imagines the two women comparing notes about their experiences in analysis, noting:

Jackson had felt that she was a "special" patient of Freud's—she was one of three patients he took to Berlin in 1930 and was the one he took to Grundlsee in September 1930. Jackson may not have gotten a kiss from Freud, but she settled for puppy love, and as a gift he gave her Fo, one of his chow Jofi's offspring.

(p. 9)

Not only were the connections between Freud and Jackson, and Thompson, and Ferenczi intense, but those between Thompson, Severn, de Forest, and Lowell were equally powerful and deserve to be more fully explored. Jackson's wish to be Freud's favorite patient and Freud's gift to her are not frequently discussed in our analytic literature, nor are the competitive feelings between Thompson, who wished to meet Freud, and Ferenczi, who kept her from meeting him. We do know that the two friends Thompson and Jackson discussed the nuances of their analytic treatments while the friendship between Freud and Ferenczi became attenuated.

Elizabeth Severn

Elizabeth Severn (1879–1959), born Leota Loretta Brown, in Milwaukee, Wisconsin, is a controversial person. Severn held no advanced degrees, but she did take classes at the Armour Institute, Chicago. She married Charles K. Haywood in 1898. Her daughter Margaret was born in 1901. Severn changed her name several times and became a healer. She was in analysis with Smith Ely Jelliffe, then Joseph Jefferson Asch, and Otto Rank, before beginning treatment with Ferenczi in 1925 (see Rachman, 2017, for greater detail).

Rachman (2017) notes that Ferenczi in two papers gave Elizabeth Severn (patient R. N.) credit for "her discoveries" during what he thought of as his "grand experiment" (p. 24). There, Ferenczi referred to her as "our colleague" who was making contributions to her own analysis and from whom he was learning how best to treat her. Rachman concludes that "It is the analysis between Ferenczi and Severn that gave birth to his pioneering ideas about trauma" (p. 25). Rachman (2014) also suggests that it was Severn who pushed Ferenczi to extend the empathic method to its farthest reaches by incorporating the analyst's personality as integral to the analytic process (p. 373).

Counting the number of times Severn is discussed in Ferenczi's *Clinical Diary*, Rachman (2017), finds that there are more references to Severn than anyone else. One of the three books Severn published, *The Discovery of the Self* (1933), grew directly out of her collaboration with Ferenczi and underscores the humanity of the analyst:

> Certain it is that unless these two people (analyst and patient) who come together for a common purpose, which is the solving of the

difficulties of the patient, can meet on equal ground, plus a lenient, sympathetic and completely unselfish attitude from the analyst no great good can be hope for.

(p. 61)

Advances in mutuality in the analytic relationship including the need for clinical empathy and the lasting effects of trauma can be attributed to Elizabeth Severn and Ferenczi as collaborators.

In her 1952 interview with Eissler, Elizabeth Severn made clear that she needed to be a clinical partner in her analysis (Rachman, 2017; Rudnytsky, 2022). She reported to Eissler that she could not tolerate any analysis that did not respect her intelligence and clinical abilities. Her analysis with Ferenczi created a democratic attitude in the clinical interaction. Severn was dubbed the "evil genius" by Freud, but in contrast, Rachman (2017) considers her to be an "iconic case" (p. 272) in psychoanalysis, equal in importance to that of Dora because it illuminated theoretical and clinical knowledge. Dora "was not helped to untie her tongue in her analysis, because her trauma experiences were not deemed significant data in the analysis" (p. 280). Severn, on the other hand, contributed to the content and direction of the analysis. She made contributions to Ferenczi's theoretical and clinical innovations between 1928 and 1933, the same period in which Clara Thompson, Izette de Forest, and Alice Lowell were his analysands. This pioneering community of analysts may seem today to have violated important analytic boundaries but in these early days of psychoanalysis they were part of a group of enthusiastic analytic supporters who dedicated themselves to developing and advancing the psychoanalytic tradition. Their contributions widened the scope of psychoanalysis to include new perspectives that we utilize in contemporary psychoanalysis—whether it is relational, interpersonal, or intersubjective.

As reported by Rachman (2017), Ferenczi acknowledged Severn contributed to his understanding of clinical empathy, non-interpretative measures, the role of childhood trauma, and mutuality. Before this pioneering innovation, a patient was considered a disturbed individual "who needed to be treated by a physician who had the superior knowledge, training, and clinical experience to provide the necessary diagnosis and therapy for their emotional problems" (p. 281). The change in status, control, and power that Severn demanded and Ferenczi allowed completely altered the clinical model.

Countess Sigray (S. I.) had previously been a patient of Elizabeth Severn before her analysis with Ferenczi. The Countess helped to pay Severn's bill to Ferenczi, enabling her to continue her analysis. Countess Sigray's sister and her brother-in-law, James Gerard, the American ambassador to Germany, socialized with Elizabeth Severn and her daughter Margaret. Brennan (2015b) points out that Severn was "upset that Countess Sigray had learned of her financial difficulties, and had paid for the rest of her analysis" (p. 11). This unexpected move humiliated Severn. An entry in the *Diary* confirms that patient R. N. is having financial trouble and help comes from an unexpecting source (Dupont, 1988). In Severn's interview with Eissler, she insinuates that Ferenczi was not charging the Countess but continued to charge Thompson, who also struggled financially (Brennan, 2015b). This may have been Severn's distortion, as Ferenczi makes no mention of not charging S. I. (Countess Sigray). Ferenczi had a very close relationship with the Countess, and in his last days, he sent for the countess along with Clara Thompson and Mrs. Vilma Kovács.

Berman (2015) finds that the triangle between Ferenczi, Elizabeth Severn (R. N.), and Hattie Sigray (S. I.) has yet to be explored. Hattie Sigray had been Elizabeth Severn's patient. In the *Diary*, Ferenczi writes: "The second person by whom [Sigray] feels persecuted possesses . . . "psychic" qualities{Severn}. Indeed, the patient has learned from the person herself that she has the power to make people do what she wants, by means of her will" (Dupont, 1988, p. 59). Sigray warned Ferenczi "against excessive self-sacrifice" (p. 46); he said she warned him "not to let myself be 'gobbled-up' by my patients" (p. 60). This probably was the source of Ferenczi's concern about "being excessively influenced by any one patient" (p. 34); in the same entry, he describes how the situation "becomes difficult when the two analysands know each other, particularly when the one I let myself be analyzed by Severn has neurotic traits and weaknesses of character that make [her] seem inferior in the eyes of the world" (p. 34).

The correspondence between de Forest and Thompson speaks to a level of intimacy and trust in their relationship. Jackson's professional history was inconsistent. She practiced psychoanalysis until 1947 and maintained her membership in American psychoanalytic organizations, serving on the editorial board of the journal *Psychoanalytic Study of the Child*. Her major contributions were in pediatric practices. She is known for changing the field of newborn hospital care, making certain that mothers and infants are roomed together (Silberman, 1998). Perhaps in her work, she vicariously rejoined the mother she lost to suicide. Problematic mothers were something Edith Jackson and Clara Thompson shared.

Alice Lowell switched her interests from psychoanalysis to internal medicine, rising to the position of Medical Director and Chief of Medicine. She was also in a same-sex relationship during a period of extreme social disapproval. In her work with Ferenczi, she found a confidence that sustained her.

Clara Thompson became a leader in the field, contributing to clinical theory and training generations of analysts after her (see, Clara M. Thompson's Professional Evolution and Legacy).

Archaeological Errors

We need to keep in mind in interpreting these interconnecting relationships to not fall prey to "confusing the map with the territory" (Levenson, 1978, p. 576). When Ferenczi talks of love, he means a deep caring, caretaking love, not a Freudian lustful instinctual love. As Severn said in her Eissler interview, Ferenczi's meaning of love was a mother's love of her child (see Rachman, 2017). It is non-erotic affection.

In a not too dissimilar vein, when Freud gives Jackson a ring and a puppy, is it a sign of affection or a boundary violation? When Jackson and Martin Freud become "attached," is it a deep friendship or a marital betrayal? When Freud tells Edith Jackson about other patients, is that a breach in confidentiality or a "consultation?" When Jackson and Irmarita Putnam "make a fully comprehensive comparison" of their analyses with Freud with Freud's approval, is that different from when Thompson and Jackson compare their treatments and Jackson tells Freud?

These events happened in a different time and culture. Boundary crossings can be benign and helpful but violations that are harmful or exploitative of the patient are transgressions.

Themes of Gender and Sexuality

Woven through many of these stories are themes of bisexuality and homosexuality, leading one colleague to ask, "Was everyone gay?" The analysts of this era were trying to understand human sexual behavior under the scientific premise of what is "normal." Anthropologists were floating the idea that culture shaped behavior and categories of gender, sex, and sexuality were culturally influenced.

In the notation for June 14, 1932, Ferenczi notes: "'Men don't understand.' Women say and are (even in analysis) very reticent about their homosexual feelings. 'Men think women can only love the possessors of penises' . . . (B, and Ett., Dm. and women friends)" (Dupont, 1988, pp. 124–125). Ferenczi reaches for a Freudian trope to understand these expressions of love, gender, sexuality, and feminism and relies on preoedipal gendered relations:

> They continue to long for a mother and female friend, with whom they can talk about their heterosexual experiences without jealousy. They prefer effeminate (passive, homosexual) men, because these offer them a continuation of bisexuality.
>
> (pp. 124–125)

These thoughts, which appear in the *Clinical Diary* under the heading "Normális feminin homosexualitás," shed light on how Alice Lowell, Izette de Forest, and Clara Thompson were struggling with the influence of patriarchy on psychoanalytic theories and society. They were reluctant to speak their true feelings to their analyst for fear of being misunderstood or pathologized. Ferenczi listens but does not hear their growing feminist understanding of gender and sexuality.

He continues to reflect on the issues under the title of "the renunciation of homosexuality": "Repression occurs at the time of first menstruation—when Tom-Boy-ishness is suppressed all of a sudden" (Dupont, 1988, p. 125). He references Dm.'s demands for him to be a mother to her and her friend Teddy. Thompson is not bound by stereotypical ideas of gender, and Ferenczi struggles to be flexible as she asks emphatically:

> "I am to overcome my ambition to be greater than he, content myself with a passive role in relation to him?"
>
> (p. 125)

Ferenczi contemplates her question and muses, "but at the same time [I must] accept her tom-boy love. Only then will she permit herself to cut herself loose from her dependence on me" (p. 125).

Thompson wants Ferenczi to accept her on her terms. He understands her request as "tom-boy love" and concedes that his patient needs this from him in order to be released from her dependency on him.

On August 4, 1932, he acknowledges: "The ease with which (Freud) sacrifices the interests of women in favor of male patients is striking. This is consistent with the unilaterally androphile orientation of his theory of sexuality" (Dupont, 1988, p. 187). For Freud, loving men was the only possibility for women. Ferenczi goes on to say that

> in this he (Freud) was followed by almost all of his pupils, myself not excluded. My theory of genitality may have good points, yet in its mode of presentation and its historical reconstruction it clings too closely to the words of the master; a new edition would mean complete rewriting.
>
> (p. 187)

These statements challenge psychoanalytic theory as it was conceived. Ferenczi suggests that the "castration theory of femininity" may need rethinking. He notes, "the author [either himself and Freud or both] may have a personal aversion to the spontaneous "female-oriented sexuality in women: idealization of the mother" (p. 188).

This auspicious feminist ending of the Clinical Diary as it relates to Clara Thompson confirms Thompson was ahead of her time in her understanding of sex and gender. It also again speaks to the importance of the personality of the analyst as well as the patient in psychoanalysis. Ferenczi and Thompson went as far as they could together. If he had lived longer they might have accomplished a "complete rewriting" of psychoanalytic theories and practices. As it turns out, she did bring back Ferenczi's ideas as she triumphantly wrote in Thompson (1955):

> Once again I have the very great pleasure of introducing the writings of Ferenczi to American readers . . . the most significant papers in this collection, the first thirteen, were written during the years of my own personal association with Ferenczi as his pupil."[3]
>
> (Thompson, 1955, p. 3)

Clara Thompson told her friend Izette de Forest in a letter on February 26, 1933, "for the first time I really feel equal to New York and all its antagonisms, and having you and Alice there will certainly make it very pleasant . . . so we'll roll up our sleeves to go to it" (Brennan, 2009, p. 448).

Thompson's analysis freed her to work hard and fight hard. Her life in New York was filled with close and influential relationships. She became an active force in organizational psychoanalysis, establishing training institutes and promoting a new form of psychoanalysis, Interpersonal Psychoanalysis.

Endings

This story of Clara Thompson's life and work presented an opportunity to hear directly from Clara Thompson about her experiences. Beginning with the interview with Kurt Eissler, it laid out the framework for an understanding of Thompson's leading role in the history of psychoanalysis. This first volume of the biography was developed in the tradition of an oral history, drawing on interviews, letters, and Thompson's essays to find the voice of Clara Thompson. There are biographical facts that inform the narrative; where Thompson was born, who her parents were, the Free Will Baptist religious community in which she was immersed during her early life. There are the competing morality themes of the times regarding the role of women in society, and Thompson's personal struggle to find a place for herself that respected her ambitions and her ethics. Thompson had a stellar education at top schools from high school through college and medical school. She won honors in her academic performance. Her love of learning guided her life. She was liked and respected by her peers but she was increasingly unhappy. Her abusive and harsh mother left her feeling unloved. In college, she broke with her mother and was estranged for nearly twenty years. She struggled with the wish to please others and her growing desire for self-actualization.

Thompson was a 20th-century woman born at a pivotal transitional time in history: white women secured the right to vote and to be educated, and gained admission to the professions. It gave her access to train with the best minds in psychiatry. She was influenced by her friendships with other colleagues interested in psychoanalysis.

She sought out psychoanalytic therapy with the quirky Snake Thompson but found it lacking. She then chose Sándor Ferenczi as her psychoanalyst because he embraced what she was looking for in an analyst—someone willing to get involved with her struggle to find psychic freedom on a deep level. It was transformative. She found her voice.

During her time in Budapest, she discovered a group of like-minded women, some of whom became friends for life. Their overlapping relationships led to both competition and intimacies. The Budapest years were a laboratory for a new psychoanalysis. Her collaboration with Ferenczi's experimental innovations put her on course to advance a new American tradition in psychoanalysis, Interpersonal Psychoanalysis.

This narrative began at the end of Thompson's career with her interview for the Freud Archives. That interview introduces the esteemed leader of Interpersonal Psychoanalysis, a woman who traveled from an oppressive religious family in pursuit of psychic freedom. *Clara M. Thompson's Professional Evolution and Legacy: An American Psychoanalyst (1933–1958)* continues the narrative of Thompson's life as she becomes a psychoanalytic pioneer and leader. This story ends at just the beginning.

Notes

1 D'Ercole, A., & Waxenberg, B. (1999). Beyond the feminine ideal: The body speaks. In M. Dimen & A. Harris (Eds.), *Storms in her head*. Other Press; D'Ercole, A. (1999). Designing the lesbian subject: Looking backwards, looking forwards. In R. Lesser and E. Schoenberg (Eds.), *That obscure subject of desire: An interdisciplinary study of Freud's female homosexual*. Routledge Press.

   Ferenczi's patient, Michael Balint, later wrote about the phenomenon as "the basic fault" (1992).

2 The relationship between Fromm, de Forest, and Thompson has not yet received sufficient attention.

3 Those first thirteen papers include "The Elasticity of Psycho-Analytic Technique" (1928), "The Principles of Relaxation and Neo-catharsis" (1930), and "Confusion of Tongues Between Adults and the Child" (1933).

References

Aron, L. (2013). *A meeting of minds: Mutuality in psychoanalysis*. The Analytic Press.

Balint, M. (1992). *The basic fault: Therapeutic aspects of regression*. Northwestern University Press.

Berman, E. (2015). On "polygamous analysis". *American Journal of Psychoanalysis*, 75(1), 29–36.

Brennan, B. W. (2009). Ferenczi's forgotten messenger: The life and work of Izette de Forest. *American Imago*, 66(4), 427–455.

Brennan, B. W. (2011). On Ferenczi: A response—From elasticity to the confusion of tongues and the technical dimensions of Ferenczi's approach. *Psychoanalytic Perspectives*, *8*(1), 1–21.

Brennan, B. W. (2015a). Out of the archive/Unto the couch: Clara Thompson's analysis with Ferenczi. In A. Harris & S. Kuchuck (Eds.), *The legacy of Sándor Ferenczi: From ghost to ancestor* (pp. 77–95). Routledge.

Brennan, B. W. (2015b). Decoding Ferenczi's clinical diary: Biographical notes. *American Journal of Psychoanalysis*, *75*(1), 5–18.

Brennan, B. W. (2018). Ferenczi's patients and their contribution to his legacy. In A. Dimitrijević, G. Cassullo, & J. Frankel (Eds.), *Ferenczi's influence on contemporary psychoanalytic traditions: Lines of development—Evolution of theory and practice over the decades* (pp. 85–97). Routledge.

de Forest, I. (1942). The therapeutic technique of Sándor Ferenczi. *International Journal of Psychoanalysis*, *23*, 120–139.

de Forest, I. (1954). *Leven of love: A development of the psychoanalytic theory and technique of Sándor Ferenczi.* Harper & Bros.

Drescher, J. (1998). I'm your handyman: A history of reparative therapies. *Journal of Homosexuality*, *36*(1), 19–42.

Drescher, J. (2008). A history of homosexuality and organized psychoanalysis. *Journal of American Academy of Psychoanalysis*, *36*(3), 443–460.

Dupont, J. (Ed.). (1988). *The clinical diary of Sándor Ferenczi* (M. Balint & N. Z. Jackson, Trans.). Harvard University Press.

Falzeder, E. (2019). *Psychoanalytic filiations: Mapping the psychoanalytic movement.* Routledge.

Ferenczi, S. (1928). The elasticity of psycho-analytic technique in M. Balint (Ed.) Final contributions to the problems & methods of psycho-analysis. pp. 87–101. Basic Books, New York 1950.

Ferenczi, S. (1930). The principles of relaxation and new-catharsis in M. Balint (Ed.) Final contributions to the problems & methods of psycho-analysis. pp. 108–125. Basic Books, New York 1950.

Ferenczi, S. (1933). Confusion of tongues between adults and the child. in M. Balint (Ed.) Final contributions to the problems & methods of psycho-analysis.pp. 156–167. Basic Books, New York 1950.

Rachman, A. W. & Klett, S. A (2019). *Analysis of the incest trauma: Retrieval, recovery, renewal.* Routledge.

Levenson, E. (1978). A perspective on responsibility. *Contemporary Psychoanalysis*, *14*, 571–578.

Lukacs, J. (1988). *Budapest 1900: A historical portrait of a city and its culture.* Grove Press.

Lynn, D. J. (2003). Freud's psychoanalysis of Edith Banfield Jackson, 1930–1936. *Journal of the American Academy of Psychoanalysis and Dynamic Psychiatry*, *31*(4), 609–625.

Rachman, A. W. (1997). *Sándor Ferenczi: The psychotherapist of tenderness and passion.* Jason Aronson.

Rachman, A. W. (2014). Sándor Ferenczi's analysis with Elizabeth Severn: "Wild analysis" or pioneering treatment of the incest trauma? *Psychoanalytic Inquiry*, *34*(2), 145–168.

Rachman, A. W. (2017). *Elizabeth Severn: The "evil genius" of psychoanalysis.* Routledge.

Rudnytsky, P. (2022). *Mutual analysis: Ferenczi, Severn, and the origins of trauma theory.* Routledge Press.

Roazen, P. (1975). *Freud and his followers.* Da Capo Press.

Roazen, P. (1995). *How Freud worked: First-hand accounts of patients.* Jason Aronson.

Severn, E. (1933). *The discovery of the self.* Rider.

Shapiro, S. A. (1993). Clara Thompson: Ferenczi's messenger with half a message. In L. Aron & A. Harris (Eds.), *The legacy of Sándor Ferenczi* (pp. 159–174). The Analytic Press.

Silberman, S. L. (1998). Edith B. Jackson, MD. *Psychoanalytic Review, 85*(1), 95–103.

Thompson, C. (1941). The role of women in this culture. *Psychiatry, 4*(1), 1–8.

Thompson, C. (1943). "The therapeutic technique of Sándor Ferenczi": A comment. *International Journal of Psychoanalysis, 24*, 64–66.

Thompson, C. (1955). Introduction. In M. Balint (Ed.), *Final contributions to the problems and methods of psychoanalysis: The selected papers of Sándor Ferenczi* (Vol. 3, p. 3). Basic Books.

Tsuruta, M. (2005) Ferenczi's footprints at the New School. The New School Bulletin, 3(2), p. 123–127.

Vass, I. (1959). Clara Thompson memorial. *The Newsletter of the White Institute, 7*(1).

Index

Note: Page numbers in *italics* indicate a figure on the corresponding page. Page numbers followed by "n" indicate a note.

For Product Safety Concerns and Information please contact our EU
representative GPSR@taylorandfrancis.com
Taylor & Francis Verlag GmbH, Kaufingerstraße 24, 80331 München, Germany